Contents

Erectile Dysfunction & Related Disorders

William Alexander
Metabolic Unit, Western General Hospital,
Edinburgh, UK

Culley Carson
Division of Urology, University of North Carolina,
Chapel Hill, North Carolina, USA

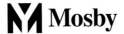
 Mosby

MOSBY
An imprint of Elsevier Limited.

The
Publisher's
policy is to use
**paper manufactured
from sustainable forests**

© 2003 Elsevier Limited.

NA Mosby is a registered trademark of Elsevier Limited.

ISBN 0-7234-3327-5

Cataloguing in Publication Data
Catalogue records for this book are available from the US Library of Congress and the British Library.

Note
Medical knowledge is constantly changing. As new information becomes available, changes in treatment, procedures, equipment and the use of drugs become necessary. The editors/authors/contributors and the publishers have taken care to ensure that the information given in this text is accurate and up to date. However, readers are strongly advised to confirm that the information, especially with regard to drug usage, complies with the latest legislation and standards of practice.

Printed by Grafos S.A. Arte sobre papel, Spain.

Abbreviations

ACE	angiotensin-converting enzyme
ADAM	androgen deficiency of the ageing male
AFUD	American Foundation for Urologic Disease
CAD	coronary artery disease
cAMP	cyclic adenosine monophosphate
cGMP	cyclic guanosine monophosphate
CNS	central nervous system
ED	erectile dysfunction
FSH	follicle-stimulating hormone
LH	luteinizing hormone
MET	metabolic equivalent of the task
MI	myocardial infarction
MUSE	medicated urethral system for erection
NO	nitric oxide
NOS	nitric oxide synthase
PDE	phosphodiesterase
PDEI	phosphodiesterase inhibitors
PVN	paraventricular nucleus
PGE_1	prostaglandin E_1
PSA	prostate-specific antigen
REM	rapid eye movement
SCA	sickle cell anaemia
SSRI	selective serotonin reuptake inhibitor
VIP	vasoactive intestinal polypeptide
VTD	vacuum tumescence device

Introduction

Sexual function has always been an area of taboo that men have been reluctant to discuss and healthcare professionals equally embarrassed to address. Impotence, or erectile dysfunction (ED), which is currently the preferred term, has been a problem for men since the beginning of time. It has until recently mainly been thought to be associated with evil and magic, and often dealt with by theologians and mystics. The term "impotence" is considered to be pejorative now that the problem is better understood and "erectile dysfunction" better covers the broad and often complex issues of disturbed male sexual function.

Serious interest amongst the medical profession started in the 20th century and initially the emphasis was predominantly on psychological issues. However, it is now recognized that there are significant physical causes in the majority of older men as well as important psychological factors, and these can now be identified and treated successfully in most cases.

Millions of men in all countries of the world suffer from ED. To some it is accepted as a natural consequence of age and is not a major problem, but in many it causes much distress to them, their relationships, and their self-esteem and social functioning.

Although ED is indeed related to age, it is also particularly common in certain important medical conditions (e.g. diabetes and cardiovascular diseases) and may be the first presenting symptom of such illnesses. It should therefore always be taken seriously and investigated and assessed as seriously as any other medical complaint.

With our current knowledge about the condition and now that successful treatments are available, it is important that all healthcare professionals both in hospitals and the community are aware of the condition and its management.

It is particularly important that primary care physicians and specialists dealing with conditions with a high prevalence of ED take on some responsibility for ED management of their patients. Recommended investigations are not complicated and initial management is now usually medical rather than of a surgical nature.

It should be emphasized that ED, whether its cause is predominantly physical or not, will not only affect the man, but also others involved in relationships. Psychological factors will always be present even if they are not the primary cause and will need discussion. Partners will also usually need to be involved if maximum benefit is to be achieved from treatment. In this respect, primary care teams of doctors and nurses may be the most appropriate people to initiate an assessment and management programme.

This rapid reference book aims to provide a clear and concise summary of current understanding, assessment and management of this important condition.

Definition

Impotence was the term most commonly used in the past. In a sexual context, impotence meant the inability of a man to achieve or sustain an erection or orgasm. In a general context, it means powerless and lacking strength. Together, this means the inability to function sexually and also generally as a man. Clearly, this is a serious problem if you happen to be male and it is no wonder that men become depressed when afflicted with the condition. Because of these rather pejorative implications it is now generally accepted that the term "erectile dysfunction" (ED) is to be preferred.

Erectile dysfunction may be defined as "the inability to obtain or maintain an erection sufficient for sexual satisfaction".

Epidemiology

The prevalence of ED of some degree in the general male population is estimated to be approximately 10%. This will vary according to culturally accepted norms and changing expectations. In the past, men generally considered discussing their sexual function to be taboo and would suffer in silence. Now that sexuality is more openly discussed and indeed publicized, expectations have increased. Such expectations have been further increased by the publicity, accessibility and success of modern treatments.

It may be therefore that more than 20 million men in the US suffer from ED. In the UK, the Impotence Association Survey (1998) suggested that 2–3 million men in the UK have significant problems from ED and that only a minority had received any worthwhile treatment.[1]

Sexual function decreases and the prevalence of ED undoubtedly increases with age. In 1948, the Kinsey report in the UK suggested the prevalence of ED to be 5% in 40-year-old men, 10% in 60-year-old men and 20% in 70-year-old men.[2] More recently, the Massachusetts Male Ageing Study suggested a similar rate, for complete erectile failure, of 9.6% in men aged 40–70 years, 5% in men aged 40 years and 15% in men aged 70 years; 25.2% of men aged 40–70 years suffered from moderate ED and 17.2% from minimal problems.[3] There is also some evidence that more sexually active men maintain better sexual function with ageing. Sexual function will of course partly depend upon the man's partner's sexual function, although satisfaction from self-stimulation may remain or become an increasingly important need.

Quality of life issues

Many, but not all, men require normal sexual function for self-confidence, self-esteem and general quality of life. They may need sexual activity to retain their feeling of masculinity. ED can therefore have a significant effect on quality of life and this may also affect their partner. Successful treatment can reverse these adverse effects.

Some adverse psychological effects of ED are listed in Table 1.

The incidence and prevalence of ED also increases with the advent or presence of concomitant disease, particularly

Table 1. Quality of life and ED
Overall quality of life of patient and partner may be adversely affected
Anxiety
Irritability and anger
Depression
Loss of self-esteem and self-confidence
Social isolation
Guilt
Partner rejection
Successful treatment can improve psychological well-being

conditions such as diabetes, cardiovascular disease, neurological conditions, urological interventions and certain medications.

Risk factors also include hypertension, smoking, dyslipidaemia and excess alcohol consumption. General psychological disturbance is also important, as are partner and relationship problems.

Aetiology

Historically, ED was considered in the mid-20th century to be predominantly a psychogenic disorder and treated as such.[4] The subsequent increased interest in the subject from urologists and other specialists in organic disease then suggested that ED was actually predominantly due to organic/physical causes. It is probably due to a combination of psychological and physical causes, with psychological factors predominating in younger (under 40 years) men and physical factors in older men.

Some important conditions associated with ED are shown in Table 2.

Table 2. Conditions associated with ED

Penile disorders	Neurological disease
Peyronie's disease	Multiple sclerosis
Trauma	Spinal injury or tumour
Congenital abnormalities	Stroke
	Multiple system atrophy
	Peripheral and autonomic neuropathy

Psychological disorders	Endocrine disease
Sexual performance anxiety	Diabetes mellitus
Sexual abuse	Hypopituitarism
Partner problems	Hypogonadism
Depression	Thyroid dysfunction
Psychoses	Hyperprolactinaemia

Cardiovascular disease	Miscellaneous
Coronary artery disease	Smoking
Stroke	Drug abuse
Peripheral vascular disease	Chronic renal failure
Multiple vascular risk factors	Rheumatoid arthritis and collagen diseases
Hypertension	Chronic debility of any cause
Type 2 diabetes	Pelvic surgery/radiotherapy
Trauma	

The pathophysiology is described later, but basically an erection is produced and sustained by a neurovascular process under central control. This process requires integrity not only of the general vascular and neurological pathways, but also specifically the ability of the penile corpora-cavernosal smooth muscle to relax and allow sufficient vascular inflow to produce erection and veno-occlusion to sustain it. Any condition or medical intervention that interferes with such a process may therefore lead to ED. Such conditions include the following.

- *Diabetes mellitus.* The overall prevalence of ED in men with diabetes is approximately 30%.[5] This increases further with age such that greater than 60% of men with diabetes aged over 60 years may be affected. In type 1 (insulin-dependent) diabetes, ED is related, like other microvascular complications, to the duration and degree of control of the condition. Diabetes is a condition that leads to premature ageing. This may be particularly true of collagen, smooth muscle and endothelial cell function. Thus, corpora cavernosal erectile tissue may be particularly unresponsive in long-standing diabetes and hence the often disappointing response of diabetic men to first- and second-line treatments. Neural integrity may be disturbed by neuropathy and vascular flow by atherosclerosis. Peyronie's disease is common in diabetes. Type 2 diabetes combines the above problems with increased cardiovascular risk factors and cardiovascular disease and this, together with age, explains the particularly high prevalence of ED.
- *Cardiovascular disease and its risk factors*. The association of cardiovascular disease and ED is important both aetiologically and therapeutically, and is discussed further later. The classic risk factors for cardiovascular disease are also associated and are listed in Table 3. ED may the first sign of occult vascular disease and a cardiovascular risk assessment should always be carried out in older men presenting with ED. The effects of cardiovascular disease and risk factors may be related directly to altered blood flow from arteriosclerosis or indirectly due to endothelial cell dysfunction. ED is common after stroke and myocardial infarction. In many such men there was probably a pre-existing problem

Table 3. Major cardiovascular risk factors associated with ED
Smoking
Hypertension
Dyslipidaemia
Family history
Diabetes

exacerbated by the physical and psychological effects of such major events. The issue of sexual function should be addressed early after such events and should be an integral part of rehabilitation. Hypertension is associated with a high prevalence of ED and debate continues as to how much is related to the hypertension itself and how much antihypertensive drug therapy contributes.

- *Depression and anxiety and other psychological disorders*. Depression and anxiety can cause erectile failure by suppressing central mechanisms and libido. Effects may vary from person to person and may be both precipitating and perpetuating factors for ED. Psychotropic drugs may also be relevant.

- *Neurological disease.* There is a strong association between some neurological disorders and ED. Clearly, if neural integrity is disrupted at any significant level ED may occur. Spinal injuries and tumours and multiple sclerosis are the most obvious examples.

- *Penile abnormalities*. Congenital or traumatic conditions. Peyronie's disease. Surgery.

- *Urological interventions.* Surgical procedures that affect the pelvic or penile nerve or blood supply, or that damage the corpora cavernosa themselves may cause ED. Radiotherapy may have a similar effect. The treatment of prostate cancer is particularly relevant in this context.

Table 4. Endocrine disorders associated with ED
Primary hypogonadism – Klinefelters, castration, orchitis
Secondary hypogonadism – Pituitary tumour, prolactinoma, hypopituitarism
Haemochromatosis
Thyroid disease – Hypothyroidism, hyperthyroidism
Diabetes mellitus
Exogenous hormone treatment/exposure

- **Chronic diseases.** Other chronic debilitating diseases may be associated with ED. The cause may be both organic or psychological. Such conditions include chronic arthritis and chronic renal failure. The prevalence of ED in men on haemodialysis may be particularly high and may be improved with renal transplantation.
- **Endocrine disease**. Endocrine diseases, particularly pituitary dysfunction and hypogonadism, are associated with sexual dysfunction (Table 4). Hyperprolactinaemia and low testosterone levels lead mainly to a primary loss of libido, leading to secondary ED.
- **Drugs.** Many drugs have been implicated in the causation of ED. Examples are listed in Table 5. It is sometimes difficult to separate the relative importance of the drug itself from the disease for which it is being used in determining the exact cause of the ED. Hypertension is a prime example. Changing drugs is probably only worthwhile if the man is sure there is a close temporal effect between the onset of ED and the taking of a particular drug. Many men will have tried stopping certain agents themselves in this respect. Drugs may exert this unwanted effect by influencing hormonal function or the central or peripheral pathways required for erectile function.

Table 5. Drugs that may be associated with ED

Antihypertensives	Drugs of abuse
Thiazide diuretics	Alcohol
Beta-blockers	Tobacco
Calcium channel blockers	Marijuana
Centrally acting: methyldopa, clonidine	Amphetamines
Ganglion blockers	Anabolic steroids
	Barbiturates
	Opiates
Antidepressants and psychotropic drugs	**Miscellaneous**
Tricyclics	Cimetidine
Monoamine oxidase inhibitors	Digoxin
Phenothiazines	Metoclopamide
Benzodiazepines	Statins
Lithium	Spironolactone
Haloperidol	
Hormones	
Oestrogens	
Anti-androgens	
Luteinizing hormone-releasing hormone analogues	

Summary

Erectile dysfunction is a common and important problem to many men. It is associated with many other medical conditions and clinicians should be aware of these associations as they may be occult and need dealing with in their own right.

Anatomy and Pathophysiology of Erectile Dysfunction

During the last 20 years, the understanding of the physiology and molecular biology of erection and erectile dysfunction (ED) has produced significant progress in the diagnosis and ultimately the treatment of men with ED. Basic science laboratory investigation has elucidated the anatomy, physiology and pharmacology of the corpus cavernosum, as well as the neurophysiology and vascular physiology of erectile function. Similarly, the mechanism of erection and its dependence upon the neurogenic, arterial and venous systems to produce erectile rigidity continues to be studied. Investigations into smooth muscle physiology, endothelial cell function, central nervous system (CNS) control with the identification of neurotransmitters such as nitric oxide (NO) and vasoactive intestinal polypeptide (VIP) in the corpus cavernosum have led to the design, development and use of specific pharmacological agents to recreate the normal physiology of the corpus cavernosum and restore erectile function in men previously termed impotent.[6,7]

Anatomy of the penis and erectile function

The gross anatomy of the human penis consists of paired vascular cylinders called the corpora cavernosa (see Figure 1). These cylinders consist of spongy smooth muscle vascular tissue with a central cavernosal artery which supplies blood for erection. The spongy tissue is surrounded by a thick fibrous fascia known as the tunica albugenea. Surrounding the tunica albuginea is a thinner layer known as Buck's fascia, which surrounds the entire penile structures. Each corporeal body communicates with the other through a gossamer septum which is not complete at the distal penile shaft. Struts of fibrous tissue are contained

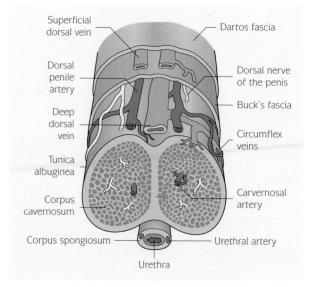

Figure 1. Cross-section of the penis.

in the corpora to provide supplemental axial rigidity. Below the corpora cavernosa is the urethra, surrounded by the corpus spongiosum. The corpus spongiosum is also a vascular structure which feeds the glans or head of the penis and provides for glans engorgement. This structure travels the length of the pendulous penis, terminating in the glans penis. Dorsal to the corpora cavernosa are the deep and superficial penile veins and the dorsal nerves of the penis. The latter supply sensation to the glans penis. The erectile tissue of the corpora consists of a lattice of vascular sinusoids surrounded by trabecular smooth muscle. Small micro-nerve endings control the functional contraction and relaxation of these smooth muscle structures. These sinusoids are lined by endothelial cells.

Vascular supply of the penis

The arterial inflow to the penis begins with the internal iliac arteries via the pudendal arterial branches (see Figure

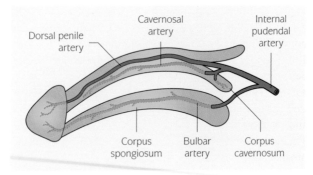

Figure 2. Arterial supply to the penis.

2). The pudendal arteries provide three branches to the penis, including the dorsal artery, paired cavernosal arteries and the bulbourethral artery. The cavernosal artery is the most important for erectile function and travels in the centre of each corpus cavernosum, giving off multiple branches called helical arteries. These in turn supply the lacunar spaces and sinusoids during erection.

Venous drainage is from the sinusoids by way of emissary veins through the tunica albuginea into the deep dorsal vein and bulbar veins. The venous drainage is ultimately to the periprostatic venous complex. The superficial dorsal vein drains the penile skin and to some degree the glans penis.

Nerve supply to the penis

Erectile function begins in the CNS close to the medial preoptic area near the hypothalamus. Many of the receptors that are present in the CNS are inhibitory and overcoming these impulses stimulates erection. The primary neurotransmitter in this area is probably dopamine in the D_2 receptors. Psychogenic erections begin with higher sensory inputs such as tactile, audiovisual or sexual fantasy stimulation associated with hormonal inputs and are relayed through the WOA to the spinal cord. Neurons in the nucleus paragigantocellularis control inhibitory impulses from the midbrain.

Spinal cord control is through the autonomic nervous system. Parasympathetic nerves from S2–S4 are the principle erectile function levels. Sympathetic input from T11–L2 controls ejaculation and detumescence. In the pelvis, these facts are combined in the pelvic plexus of nerves to form the cavernous nerves. These nerves course from anterior to the rectum, posterolateral to the prostate and into the corpora cavernosa at the base of the penis. These are the nerves which may be damaged by radical prostatectomy or colectomy.

Once in the penile tissue, the nerves control the relaxation and contraction of the lacunar smooth muscles through specific neurotransmitters. The primary nerve type is the non-adrenergic/non-cholinergic nerves. The primary neurotransmitter from these nerves is NO.

The sensory function of the penis is also controlled by these peripheral nerves, as they contain both sensory and motor components and function through a reflex arc in the lumbar spinal cord in an area known as the spinal erection centre. Reflex erections can therefore be seen in men with spinal cord disruption above the spinal cord erection centre.

Hormonal control of erectile function

It has long been known that sexual performance and interest depend upon an adequate supply of the male hormone testosterone and normal androgenic function of the pituitary gland, testicles and adrenal glands. A clearer understanding of the role of testosterone has shown that the presence of testosterone receptors in the CNS facilitate sexual functioning and that, peripherally, testosterone is responsible for full function of nitric oxide synthase (NOS) in the corpus cavernosum smooth muscle cells.[8]

The testosterone levels produced in the normal adult male begin with the hypothalamus, which produces gonadotrophin-releasing hormone that stimulates the anterior pituitary gland to produce luteinizing hormone (LH) and follicle-stimulating hormone (FSH). These latter two directly stimulate the testes; LH acts on the Leydig cells to produce testosterone from its precursor, cholesterol. Testosterone then provides feedback control to the pituitary and hypothalamus. LH and FSH are both secreted in a pulsatile fashion and testosterone is produced in a diurnal pattern, such that it is highest in the early morning and lowest in the evening. This morning peak is most pronounced in the young male and flattens as men age.

Molecular physiology of erection

For an erection to occur, the central cavernosal arteries of the corpora cavernosa must dilate to increase blood flow to the penis. This increased blood flow and the production of NO from nerve endings in the smooth muscles forming the lacunar spaces of the corpora cavernosa produces lacunar smooth muscle relaxation, decreasing outflow resistance.[6] Once smooth muscle relaxation has occurred, blood flows rapidly into the lacunar spaces, increasing the volume in the corpora cavernosa. Subsequent compression and elongation of the subtunical veins draining the corpora cavernosa is caused by the increased volume and pressure of the erectile bodies and produces decreased venous outflow and increased intracorporeal pressure. Pressure in the corpora cavernosa is supplemented by contraction of the perineal muscles, such as the bulbocavernosus and ischiocavernosus muscles, resulting in a high pressure rigid erection satisfactory for sexual activity. The pressure produced in this rigid column exceeds the pressure in the abdominal aorta.

On a subcellular level, control of smooth muscle activity is dependent upon intracellular calcium flux. Neurotransmitters and endothelium-derived factors influence the flow of intracellular calcium balancing penile flaccidity and rigidity. The principle substance responsible for smooth muscle relaxation is the neurotransmitter NO.[7] NO is produced from the precursor L-arginine through the enzyme NOS. NO subsequently diffuses into smooth muscle cells, activates the secondary neurotransmitter system guanylate cyclase, which converts guanosine triphosphate into cyclic guanosine monophosphate (cGMP). This secondary neurotransmitter activates the intracellular sodium pump system, opening potassium channels and producing a decrease in intracellular potassium and decreased intracellular calcium with resultant smooth muscle relaxation.[9] cGMP is metabolized through enzymatic breakdown by phosphodiesterase type 5 (PDE5). Once the concentrations of cGMP are low enough, smooth muscle contraction recurs from closing of potassium channels, increased intracellular calcium and smooth muscle contraction.

Other neurotransmitters involved as co-transmitters include VIP and prostaglandins, which act through the adenylate cyclase pathway and its secondary neurotransmitter cyclic adenosine monophosphate (cAMP).[10,11]

Smooth muscle relaxation is counterbalanced by neurotransmitters and substances which produce smooth muscle contraction.[12] These agents, which are present in the normal corpus cavernosum, may be increased by high sympathetic tone associated with physical and psychological stressors. The vasoconstrictor norepinephrine is the principle agent responsible for smooth muscle contraction. Norepinephrine is released from the sympathetic nerve endings in the corpora cavernosa and activates the alpha-1 adrenoceptors, raising intracellular calcium and producing smooth muscle contraction.[13] Other similar molecules may also be involved in smooth muscle contraction. These include endothelin-1, prostaglandin F_2 and epinephrine. Levels of these local neurotransmitters, as well as CNS substances which can be manipulated pharmacologically, has led to the revolution in the pharmacological treatment of ED.[14]

Summary

Erection is produced by a coordination of neurotransmitters, the principal of which is NO, stimulated by nerve transmission from the midbrain via the spinal cord and peripheral nerves. The tissue of the corpora cavernosa

Diagnosis and Assessment of Erectile Dysfunction

Ascertainment

It is important to identify the problem of ED because men with ED may be reluctant to admit to it as a problem because of embarrassment. Healthcare professionals may also be reluctant to do so because of lack of confidence in dealing with it.

Screening for high-risk patients such as those attending diabetes and cardiovascular clinics is one way of overcoming this problem. Alternatively, the obvious availability of posters and educational leaflets can be helpful. The latter will also give partners the opportunity to raise the subject and give couples the opportunity to discuss the problem in more depth.

History

A full history of the complaint is the most important part of the assessment and should include details of the sexual problem as well as of general health to identify underlying disease or risk factors. Cultural and social issues will need to be considered.

Men should be encouraged to attend with their partners when possible, but will usually attend alone. Despite this, the partner must be considered as they themselves may have significant problems.

The majority of men will have true ED with the inability to obtain or sustain an erection sufficient for sexual satisfaction. It is important, however, to define exactly what the problem is. Erectile dysfunction may be understood to include a number of other problems, both physical and psychological, and some of these are shown in Table 6.

It is important not only to establish exactly what the problem is, but also to ascertain the likely causes in order

Table 6. Problems other than ED causing sexual dysfunction

Congenital abnormalities

Penile curvature – Peyronie's disease

Balanitis and phimosis

Ejaculatory disorders

Orgasmic problems

Misconceptions of normality

Diminished or lack of libido

Psychosexual problems

Table 7. Factors discriminating between a physical and a psychological cause

Physical cause	Psychological cause
Gradual onset	Sudden onset
Persistent and consistent	Intermittent and partner variable
No spontaneous or self-stimulated erection	Spontaneous/self-stimulated erection occurs
No overt psychological problems	Overt psychological problems
Significant physical conditions	No significant physical disorder

to be able to give a reasoned explanation of the problem and explanation of possible management. A history from the partner or of the partner's attitude is also important in this respect.

It may be useful to consider whether the problem is predominantly psychological or physical. In this respect, the discriminating factors listed in Table 7 have been said to be useful.

A full medical history is also important, particularly regarding cardiovascular risk, and should also include a drug history. A sample of a clinical assessment proforma is shown in Figure 3.

Erectile failure proforma

Name . . . . Date . . . .

Address . . . .

. . . .

Post code . . . . GP . . . .

Problem

1. **Erections**: Failure obtain/sustain   Onset: Sudden/Gradual
                       Partial/Complete failure   Duration of problem:
Nocturnal Yes/No   Spontaneous Yes/No
Masturbation Yes/No   Partner Yes/No   Single Yes/No
Intercourse: Occasional/Never/Last time =
2. **Ejaculation**: Normal / Retro / Quick / None   Orgasm: Yes/No
3. **Libido**:   Normal / Reduced
4. **Relationship**:   Psychology:

Other conditions

Diabetes: NIDDM / IDDM.   Duration =   .Rx
Microvascular disease: Yes/No
Vascular: IHD: Yes/No PVD: Yes/No   CVD: Yes/No Cigs: Yes/No
Dyslipidaemia: Yes/No   Hypertension: Yes/No   Rx:
Neurological:
Psychiatric/Psychological:
Urological:
Peyronies: Yes/No

Comments:

Medications

Cause

Congenital:
Acquired: Organic / Psychological / Mixed O+P / Mixed P+0
Organic =

Examination	Penis	Testes	Prostate
Investigation	Testosterone	Total:	Androgen Index:
		Free:	DHEAs
	Prolactin		
	PSA		
	Other		

Treatment		Initial	Subsequent (date)
			1 2 3 4
	Oral		
	Vacuum device:	Type:	
	Self injection:	Type:	
	MUSE:		
	Psychosexual:		
	None:		
	Other:		

Seen by: Date: Review:

Figure 3. Clinical proforma.

Validated questionnaires are available which can be used to obtain full details of sexual function from the man and partner. Although unnecessary in routine clinical practice, they can be useful in particular circumstances and for research. Examples are shown in Appendix 4.

Standard questions that may be usefully asked include (see Table 8):

- What exactly is the problem?
  Failure to obtain/sustain an erection.
  Severity.
  Presence or absence of spontaneous or self-stimulated erection.
  Is it a different problem, e.g. ejaculatory disorder, libido problem, Peyronie's disease, etc.
  How did it start and how long has it been a problem?
- What do you think is the likely cause?
  In some men there will be a definite relationship to the onset of certain conditions or medications.
  It is worth asking whether the man thinks it is psychological or physical. It may be worth determining predisposing, precipitating, potentiating and perpetuating factors.
- Why is it a problem and what is the partner's attitude?
  Sexual function in general should be discussed and relationship issues in particular. The partner should always be invited to attend, but most men will usually attend alone initially.
- What treatments do you know about and how would you wish to proceed?
  Many men will be aware of treatments but some will have no idea at all. Some men will not wish to pursue treatments but are pleased to have been able to talk about the problem and have it explained. It is important to mention all treatment options.

Physical examination

The physical examination is important not only to help to ascertain the likely cause of ED, but also to check for other significant disease suggested by the history and finally to

Table 8. Medical history taking and ED
Standard questions that may be usefully asked: • What *exactly* is the problem?   • What do you think is the likely cause?   • Why is it a problem and what is your partner's attitude?   • What do you know about treatments and how would you like to proceed?

be sure certain physical treatments are going to be practicable and safe.

It is essential to examine the genitalia, the cardiovascular and the endocrine systems. Neurological and other systems may require examination if the history suggests relevant or significant pathology (Table 9).

The genitalia should be examined for any penile abnormalities, including size and shape, the presence of phimosis or Peyronie's disease. Testicular volume should be assessed and any other signs of possible hypogonadism sought. Signs of hypopituitarism or thyroid disease should be looked for if these conditions are suggested.

Cardiovascular examination should include measurement of blood pressure, peripheral pulses and bruits.

Table 9. Essentials of physical examination in the man with ED	
General	Hair distribution and body habitus for endocrine disease
	Gynaecomastia
	Depression and anxiety
Genitalia	Penis for size, phimosis, Peyronie's disease
Cardiovascular	Blood pressure and peripheral vasculature
Other	If suggested by history, e.g. neurological, prostate

Table 10. Investigations and ED	
Essential	Plasma glucose, HbA$_{1c}$
General	Lipid profile
	Testosterone, prolactin, LH and FSH
	Thyroid function
	Renal and liver function
	Prostate-specific antigen (PSA)
	Microbiology
Specialist	Colour Doppler imaging
	Cavernosography
	Arteriography

Investigations

The only essential laboratory investigation is to exclude diabetes and should include a venous plasma glucose and glycosylated haemoglobin estimation.

Other general investigations will depend upon the outcome of the history and examination (see Table 10), and might include:

- Lipid profile if vascular disease.
- Testosterone if reduced libido and/or hypogonadism suspected.
- Prolactin, LH and FSH if testosterone reduced.
- Thyroid function if thyroid disease suspected.
- Microbiology cultures if infection suspected.
- Prostate-specific antigen (PSA) if cancer of prostate suspected or androgen therapy considered.

Specialist investigations may be necessary if specialist surgery is anticipated.

Discussion

The final part of the assessment should be discussion of the various treatment options, their advantages and disadvantages, and relative suitability to the individual. Explanatory leaflets may be helpful for the man to discuss with his partner.

Treatment

Men should be made aware of all available treatment options. The choice will depend upon the individual man's preference, the clinician involved and the availability of the treatments.

Lifestyle

Erectile dysfunction is often associated with other conditions and particularly cardiovascular risk factors. General advice should be given regarding smoking, alcohol, weight and general fitness. This may not improve the ED, but is important generally. Such advice should not be a substitute for other treatment but given in conjunction.

Relationship issues

It is essential that the man's relationship with his partner is discussed. Simply restoring erectile function may not resolve all issues and lead to adequate sexual satisfaction. It may be helpful, particularly if there is performance anxiety, to discuss techniques such as the Masters and Johnson sensate-focusing techniques.[4] This may improve communication and understanding between partners.

Men with severely dysfunctional relationships should be referred for specialist counselling.

Table 11 outlines the currently available treatment categories. At present, oral therapy is the most satisfactory first line of action.

Psychosexual therapy

Psychological sexual dysfunction is also called psychogenic and should be a specific diagnosis and not a diagnosis of exclusion. Indeed, psychogenic ED in the presence of organic aetiologies or risk factors should be referred to as mixed ED. True psychogenic ED may be associated with couples disorders, hypoactive sexual desire disorder or

Table 11. Currently available treatments for ED

Psychosexual therapy

Topical treatments

Oral treatments and androgen replacement

Intraurethral treatment

Intracavernosal injection treatment

Vacuum tumescence devices

Surgery

depression. These underlying conditions should be identified for specific therapy as they may have a direct impact on the treatment of psychogenic ED.

Psychogenic ED may be divided into immediate and delayed types as defined by Rosen.[15] Immediate includes performance anxiety, couples or partnership disorders and inadequate stimulation. Delayed or remote types include childhood sexual trauma, identity disorders, religious and cultural issues that impact on sexual performance. Masters and Johnson were the first to bring popular attention to the issues of performance anxiety or fear of failure.[4] This "spectator" role spawned the Masters and Johnson "sensate focus method" of treatment. Indeed, arousal problems have been documented with stress, anxiety and depression. These conditions do not in themselves cause sexual dysfunction, but lead to changes in attention and perceptual processing associated with both male and female sexual dysfunction.

Couples or partner issues are also important in sexual function. Problems with communication, trust, lack of intimacy and power conflicts are associated with ED. These conflicts may be a cause or a result of sexual dysfunction and may be difficult to treat without identifying the underlying problems in the couple's interactions.

Psychogenic ED may be primary or secondary. Primary psychogenic ED is defined as lifelong with no previous satisfactory sexual function, while secondary psychogenic

ED is acquired after a period of normal or adequate sexual function. Secondary problems may be the result of medications, significant psychological pathology or lifestyle changes.[16,17] Secondary is far more frequent and is more easily resolved with treatment.[18]

Diagnosis of psychogenic ED should be made by history and physical examination. Problems with human sexuality are always associated with issues of self-esteem, relationship problems, gender and moral values and couples issues. The physician's comfort level with discussion of sexuality is critical in obtaining a good sexual history. The patient and his partner must perceive that the physician is knowledgeable but also flexible, sympathetic and confidential with their plight. The patient and partner must be placed at ease and questions while probing should be considerate of the patient's culture, background and beliefs.[19]

A careful physical examination and laboratory testing are also essential to identify organic risk factors. Questionnaires such as the SHIM for ED and Beck's Depression Inventory (BDI) may be useful in the diagnosis.[20] Laboratory studies should include a hormone profile. If suspected, a thyroid function profile may identify an occult thyroid aetiology, since both hypo- and hyperthyroidism are associated with ED.

If either physical examination or laboratory studies are abnormal, a mixed aetiology may be diagnosed. While no satisfactory testing procedures are available, some use the nocturnal penile tumescence and rigidity monitor for assistance in difficult situations.[19] The normal man should have three to six erections per night during rapid eye movement (REM) sleep and these erections should be 20–45 minutes in duration, with at least 55% tip and base cross-section rigidity. These studies may be influenced by poor sleep patterns, sleep apnoea, medications that inhibit REM sleep and anxiety.

The treatment of psychosexual disorders progresses in four areas according to Rosen.[15] Anxiety reduction and desensitization, cognitive behavioural intervention, increased sexual stimulation, and interpersonal assertiveness and couple's communication training are some of the techniques and approaches used. While these are the usual approaches, no studies have been reported to document the treatment outcomes, best approach or identification of the best method for a specific problem area.[21]

Perhaps one of the most difficult situations is that of low libido or desire, termed hypoactive sexual desire disorder. These patients should be carefully assessed to identify previous sexual dysfunction, health issues and depression. An experienced sexual counsellor best performs treatment.

Psychogenic factor sexual dysfunction may occur alone or in combination with organic factors (mixed ED).[22] The most frequent causes of this form of ED are depressed mood, low self-esteem, stress and anxiety.[15] Couple's issues are also common and interview with both partners of a couple may elucidate some of these issues.[19] Diagnosis should include careful sexual history, physical examination and laboratory studies. A nocturnal penile tumescence study may be helpful in selected patients. Once identified, traditional treatment consists of anxiety reduction, desensitization procedures, and cognitive behavioural intervention couples counselling and guided stimulation exercises. Currently, these techniques are aided by the use of oral agents to provide support and gratification during the counselling process.

Conclusions

Psychogenic risk factors for ED include anxiety, depression, low libido and performance issues.[23] Psychogenic associated ED occurs as mixed in most patients with organic risks. Treatment with psychological modalities alone is frequently unsuccessful and long-term cure rare. Combining oral ED agents and psychological counselling or treatment will have better results than either therapy alone. Patients with psychogenic associated or mixed ED should be encouraged to seek counselling in addition to their pharmacological programme.

Topical treatments

Many topical drug creams and pastes have been tried. They include smooth muscle relaxants and/or vasodilators with or without transdermal permeation enhancers.

Topical intraurethral and other methods of medication delivery may produce adequate erectile function in patients without the invasiveness of self-injection.[24,25] Topical application has included transcutaneous and urethral absorption of a variety of pharmacological agents. Minoxidil, an antihypertensive agent which produces significant arterial dilation as a potassium channel opener, has been applied topically as a 2% solution.[24] While the results of minoxidil application were superior to placebo, satisfactory rigidity was not obtained for clinical use. Nitroglycerine, an older established vasodilator, can be applied transcutaneously using an ointment formulation.[26,27] A randomized placebo-controlled double-blind trial demonstrated a significant response in patients treated with nitroglycerine patches with satisfactory erectile function in 21 of 26 patients with mild ED. Side-effects included headache and penile erythema.[27] Because topical nitroglycerine is rapidly absorbed through vaginal mucosa, patients using transcutaneous or ointment-based nitroglycerine for ED must be advised to wear a condom during sexual activity. A newer preparation of prostaglandin E_1 (PGE_1) in SEPA gel has undergone early trials.[28] McVary et al.[29] report 67–75% satisfactory erections within 60 minutes using visual sexual stimulation. More than 75% of all men (both placebo and PGE_1) reported glans discomfort.

Androgen replacement therapy

Controversy remains regarding the use of androgen replacement therapy in men with ED. In men with proven hypogonadism, it is important for the restoration of secondary sexual characteristics, muscle and bone mass, and sexual interest and behaviour.

There is not convincing evidence that it is beneficial in restoring erectile function in men with normal or slightly reduced testosterone levels.

There are theoretical risks of adverse effects on the prostate and, if used, it is recommended that PSA levels be monitored in men over the age of 50 years.

Oral therapy

Oral therapies currently include:

1. Peripherally active: Phosphodiesterase 5 (PDE5) inhibitors: Sildenafil, Tadalafil, Vardenafil.
2. Centrally active: Apomorphine.

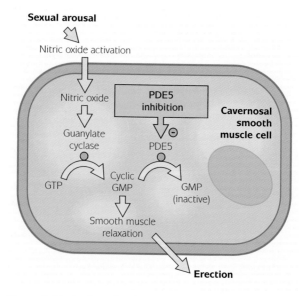

Figure 4. Mechanism of action of PDE5 inhibition. Adapted with permission from Eardley I, Sethia K. *Erectile Dysfunction: Current Investigation and Management*. London: Mosby, 2003.

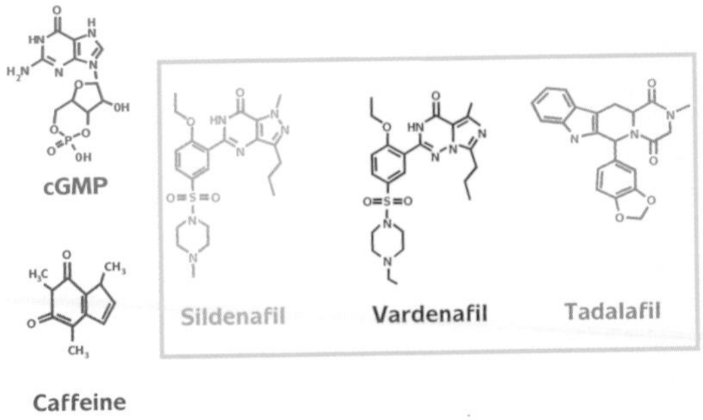

cGMP

Sildenafil Vardenafil Tadalafil

Caffeine

Figure 5. Structure of sildenafil, vardenafil and tadalafil.

Phosphodiesterase inhibitors (PDEIs)

PDE5 inhibitors act peripherally on the penile erectile smooth muscle. Inhibition of PDE5 leads to an increase in cyclic-GMP. This in turn potentiates the action of nitric oxide and thereby enhances cavernosal smooth muscle relaxation and penile erection during sexual stimulation.

Figure 4 outlines the intracellular action of PDE5 inhibitors.

There are currently three available PDE5Is: sildenafil (Viagra), tadalafil (Cialis), vardenafil (Levitra), with others under development. The structure of these drugs is shown in Figure 5.

Sildenafil (Viagra) was the first of the PDE5 inhibitors and has been hugely successful and well tried and tested. It is effective in greater than 70% of men with ED of mixed aetiologies.[30] Lower success rates of approximately 60% are found in conditions associated with particularly severe ED such as diabetes and cardiovascular disease.[31]

Tadalafil and vardenafil are likely to prove equally effective.

Vardenafil is similar in structure and effect although may be slightly quicker acting. Tadalafil has a much longer half-

Table 12. Comparison of newer PDE5 inhibitors			
	Vardenafil	**Sildenafil**	**Tadalafil**
Doses (mg)	5, 10, 20	20, 50,100	10, 20
Onset (minutes)	15–60	30–60	30–60
WOO factor*	4	4	24+
Efficacy %	60–80	60–80	60–80
Cost**	6	6	5

*Window Of Opportunity, in hours.

** £ per maximum dose/tablet.

life than the others and will have the potential advantage of a longer window of opportunity remaining active for 24–36 hours after ingestion. This may prove helpful for some men and improve spontaneity of sexual activity.

Some general comparative data are shown in Table 12 and effectiveness in Figures 6–8.

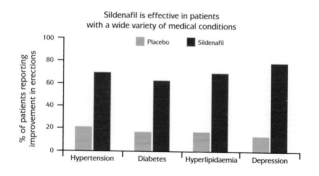

Figure 6. Effectiveness of sildenafil in patients with a variety of medical conditions.[32] Adapted from Kloner R, Brown M. Am J Hypertens 2001; 14: 70–73 and Pfizer Inc, NY - data on file.

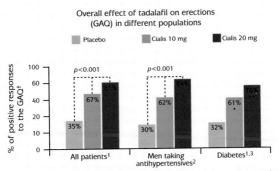

†GAQ: "Has the treatment you have been taking over the last 12 months improved your erections?"
*$p<0.01$ versus placebo; **$p<0.001$ versus placebo

Figure 7. Effect of cialis on different population Data from Brock GB *et al. J Urol* 2002; 168: 1332–1336,[33] Padmaa-Nathan H *et al.* Poster presented at ASH 2002, NY, USA and Eli-Lilly - data on file.

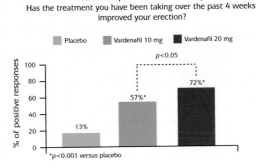

Figure 8. Vardenafil phase III diabetes study.

PDE5Is are only effective in conjunction with sexual stimulation and arousal.

Dosing should be started with the lowest dose and increased as necessary. Most patients with severe organic ED will require higher doses. Higher than recommended doses are associated with a higher incidence of side-effects.

Suggested advice for maximum efficacy of sildenafil is shown in Table 13 and prescribing advice for tadalafil and vardenafil in Tables 14 and 15.

Effectiveness depends upon an adequate trial of use. It is suggested for instance that sildenafil should be tried in adequate dosage on at least six separate occasions prior to abandoning it if ineffective.

Table 13. Suggested advice for maximal efficacy of sildenafil

Take on empty stomach for fastest effect

Avoid alcohol

Ensure adequate sexual stimulation

Sexual activity within 1–4 hours

Try adequate dosage: 100 mg if 50 mg ineffective

Try full dosage on at least six separate occasions

Table 14. How to prescribe tadalafil

Start with 10 mg and titrate to 20 mg if necessary

Taken 30 minute to 12 hours prior to sexual activity

With or without food

Sexual stimulation required

Table 15. How to take vardenafil

Dosage will be determined by response and doctor's advice

Swallow one tablet with a glass of water

Take 25–60 minutes before sexual activity

Can be taken with or without food, though preferably not after a heavy or high fat meal

Do not use more than once daily

Table 16. PDE5 inhibitors and cardiovascular disease
Well tolerated
Similar effect to nitrates
Effective in 60–80%
No effect on heart rate
No effect on ECG
Modest fall in BP—8–10SBP, 4–6DBP (6 hours)
No increased death, MI, CVA

PDE5Is are generally considered safe in men with cardiovascular disease or risk factors (see Table 16) provided that the man is fit enough for sexual activity. Their use is contraindicated in conjunction with nitrates and NO donors such as Nicorandil.

(See later section for further details regarding cardiovascular disease and ED.)

Cautions and contraindications are outlined in Table 17. Side-effects will vary depending upon the relative inhibition of other phosphodiesterases as can be seen in Table 18. For example tadalafil does not effect retinal PDE6 and therefore does not have the potential to cause visual disturbance. The visual disturbance that may occur with higher doses of sildenafil or vardenafil usually presents as a temporary blue distortion of colour vision and is not of serious consequence. Myalgia and back pain is unique to tadalafil.

Drug interactions with PDE5Is are shown in Table 19. PDE5Is undergo hepatic metabolism via cytochrome P450 CYP3A4. CYP3A4 inhibitors may therefore increase and CYP3A4 inducers reduce levels of PDE5 inhibitors.

PDE5 inhibitors are generally considered to be the first line treatment for men with organic erectile failure and

Table 17. Side-effects, cautions and contraindications with currently available PDE5 inhibitors

Side-effects

Headache

Dizziness

Flushing

Dyspepsia

Visual disturbance (s, v)

Myalgia, back pain (t)

Cautions

Renal impairment (v, s, t)

Deformities of penis(v, s, t)

Priapism risk — sickle-cell, myeloma, leukaemia (v, s, t)

Active peptic ulceration (v, s)

Elderly (>75 years) and CYP3A4 inhibitors (v)

Concomitant use of alpha blockers not recommended (v)

Contraindications

Nitrates (v, s, t)

Hereditary retinal disorder (v, s)

Recent stroke/MI (v, s, t)

Severe CVS disease—unfit for sexual activity (v, s, t)

End stage renal failure—dialysis (v)

Severe hepatic impairment (v, s)

Hereditary galactose intolerence (Lapp enzyme) (t)

v=vardenafil; s=sildenafil; t=tadalafil

sildenafil has revolutionized the management of ED by increasing awareness, acceptability and availability of effective treatment. They can also be used as an adjunct to psychosexual therapy in men with predominant psychogenic ED. The choice of PDE5I will depend upon the preference and needs of individual patients and clinicians.

Table 18. Comparisons of sildenafil, vardenafil and tadalafil PDE 1–11[34,35]

	PDE1	PDE2	PDE3	PDE4	PDE5	PDE6 (rod)	PDE6 (cone)	PDE7	PDE8	PDE9	PDE10	PDE11
					IC_{50} (nM) (Fold selectivity versus, PDE5)							
Sildenafil	280 (80)	68000 (>19000)	13200 (4628)	7200 (2057)	3.5 (--)	37 (10.5)	34 (9.7)	21300 (6100)	29800 (8500)	261 (750)	9800 (2800)	2730 (780)
Vardenafil	69 (690)	6200 (62000)	4000 (40000)	4000 (47000)	0.1 (--)	3.5 (35)	0.6 (6)	>30000 (>3000000)	>30000 (>3000000)	580 (5800)	3000 (30000)	162 (1620)
Tadalafil	<30000 (>4000)	>30000 (>4000)	>30000 (>4000)	>30000 (>4000)	6.7	1260 (188)	1030 (153)	>100000 (>14000)	>100000 (>14000)	>100000 (>4000)	>100000 (>4000)	37.0 (5.5)

Table 19. PDE5 inhibitors drug interactions

CYP3A4 inhibitors
Ketoconazole
Itraconazole
Erythromycin
Clarithromycin
Grapefruit jiuce

CYP3A4 inducers
Rifampicin
Phenobarbitone
Phenytoin
Carbamazepine

Protease inhibitors
Ritonavir, Saquinavir
Nitrates and NO donors
Antihypertensves

Apomorphine SL (Uprima)[36]

The other oral agent currently available is apomorphine. This is a sublingual preparation.

It exerts its effect centrally by stimulating the dopamine receptors in the paraventricular nucleus of the brain. Mechanisms of action are shown in Table 20. Its onset of action is within 20 minutes.

Dosage should start with 2 mg and be increased to 3 mg if necessary and tolerated. Higher doses can be used but are associated with more side-effects. Side-effects, cautions and contraindications are outlined in Table 21.

Efficacy is best in mild or psychogenic ED. It is less effective in severe cases. Some efficacy rates are shown in Table 22.

Table 20. Mechanisms of action of apomorphine

Dopamine receptor agonist

Paraventricular nucleus (PVN) and spinal cord

Release of pro-erectile neurotransmitters

Decrease anti-erectile sympathetic tone

Libido

Table 21. Side-effects, cautions and contraindications with apomorphine

Side-effects

Nausea

Yawning and somnolence

Headache

Dizziness

Syncope

Rhinitis

Taste disorder

Cautions

Nitrates

Antihypertensive treatments

Dopamine agonists/antagonists

Contraindications

Severe CVS disease

Unfit for sexual activity

Hypotension

Table 22. Some efficacy rates and cost of sublingual apomorphine for the treatment of ED

Efficacy

4 mg: 54% effective versus 33% placebo

3 mg: 47% effective versus 32% placebo

Cost

£5 per 3 mg tablet

It can be used safely in patients with cardiovascular disease and is generally safe if used with caution in combination with nitrates and other NO donors such as Nicorandil.

Intraurethral therapy

Intraurethral alprostadil is available as MUSE (medicated urethral system for erection; see Figure 9). The intraurethral application of alprostadil (PGE_1) has been demonstrated in multiple studies and through clinical practice.[29,37] A pellet containing PGE_1 is applied to the urethra through the MUSE, delivering PGE_1 to the corpus cavernosum providing smooth muscle relaxation through activation of the adenylate cycling system and reducing intracellular calcium. Phase III trial results have documented erectile function in as many as 66% of men with ED of a variety of aetiologies.[37] Doses available range from 125 to 1000 micrograms, and side-effects of treatment include urethral pain and urethral trauma. Porst[38] compared intraurethral and intracavernosal injected PGE_1 with a significantly higher success rate and decreased side-effects with injection of PGE_1 at lower doses compared with intraurethral application of PGE_1. The use of the MUSE system for oral medication failures and in selective patients with unsatisfactory erections with penile prostheses establishes a niche for this method of treatment of ED. Recent studies using a combination of the selective alpha-1 blocker

1. Open the foil pouch and allow MUSE to slide out of the pouch. Keep the pouch for disposing of the applicator after use.

2. Hold the body of the MUSE applicator, remove the protective cover by twisting, and pull the body out from the cover, **Be carefull not to push in or pull out the applicator button** and avoid touching the stem or the tip of the applicator.

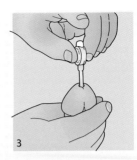

3. While **sitting** or **standing**, extend your penis gently to its full length. Taking several seconds, **slowly insert the MUSE applicator into the end of the penis up to the level of the collar.**

4. Once inserted, slowly and completely push down the ejector button and **hold the applicator in place for 5 seconds**, to release the medication inside the penis.

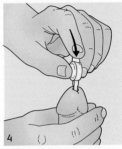

5. Gently rock the applicator to the right and left inside the penis, to make sure the pellet has been released. Gently withdraw the applicator with the penis upright.

6. Roll the penis, in an upright position and stretch to its full length, between the hands for ten seconds to distribute the medication.

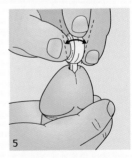

7. Replace the cover on the stem of the applicator and discard the whole thing inside the foil pouch. **Then sit, stand or walk around for 10 minutes as the erection develops.**

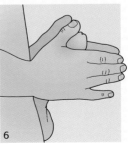

Figure 9. MUSE diagram and administration steps.

prazosin resulted in minimal but significant increase in efficacy over single drug therapy.

However, success with MUSE has been variable. Experience with men using the preparation at home has been disappointing, with a much lower success rate in men with severe organic ED.[39] Most men require the higher doses and continued use has also been limited by side-effects, particularly penile and lower extremity pain (see Table 23).

A constriction ring (Actis, see Figure 10) can be used in conjunction to reduce proximal absorption and help sustain the erection.

Patient studies have shown men to prefer self-injection therapy.[40]

Table 23. MUSE: advantages and disadvantages

Advantages	Disadvantages
Simple delivery method	Variable efficacy
No injection required	Poor efficacy in severe organic ED
	Intolerance due to penile and lower extremity pain

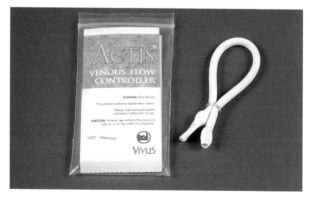

Figure 10. Constriction ring. Reproduced with permission from Vivus Corporation.

Use of a condom is also recommended to prevent transfer of prostaglandin to the partner and this is particularly important if the partner is pregnant.

Intracavernosal injection therapy

Intracavernosal injection treatment with vasoactive drugs for the treatment of ED began in 1982 after the discovery of its efficacy by Virag in France and Brindley in the UK.[41,42] Until sildenafil became available it was the treatment of first choice for most men (see Figure 11). Originally, papaverine was the drug most commonly used and if ineffective was then combined with phentolamine. It was cheap and effective but never licensed for use in the UK and was thought to be associated with a relatively high incidence of penile fibrosis and priapism if excessive doses were used.

Prostaglandin E_1 (alprostadil) is now the drug most commonly used in the UK, but its expense, shorter half-life and uncomfortable erection in some men have assured the continued use of the papaverine and phentolamine combination in some patients in Europe and the USA.[43] In

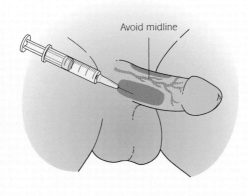

Avoid midline

Figure 11. Intracavernosal injection treatment.

patients where this two-drug combination fails to produce satisfactory erectile function, a three-drug therapy known as Trimix may salvage non-responders. This combination of papaverine, phentolamine and PGE_1 permits a reduced dosage of each agent with increased safety and decreased morbidity. Papaverine's pharmacological function occurs as a result of increasing intracellular cAMP concentrations with subsequent decrease in calcium concentration and smooth muscle relaxation of all vascular structures in the penis. Phentolamine functions through its activity as a non-selective alpha-adrenoceptor blocker, inhibiting smooth muscle contraction. PGE_1, a prostanoid, produces smooth muscle relaxation in both the corpus cavernosum and arteriolar structures in the corpus cavernosum through the cAMP pathway, decreasing intracellular calcium concentrations.[6] Satisfactory erections from injection of PGE_1 at a dose range from 5 to 40 micrograms are in excess of 70%, with prolonged erections occurring in 1% and corpus cavernosum fibrosis in only 2.7%.[43,44]

Other combinations of injectable agents are available internationally. A combination of phentolamine and VIP has been approved in several European countries.[45,46] This combination product (Invicorp, Senetec) has responses equivalent to PGE_1 without penile pain and aching.[47] Moxisylyte, a selective alpha-1 receptor blocking substance, has also been approved for use in several European countries.[48,49] This agent, which relaxes smooth muscle in a fashion similar to phentolamine, has a reported success rate of 70% at doses of 10–30 mg. Adverse events include prolonged erection (1%) and corpus cavernosum fibrosis (1.5%). Comparisons between moxisylyte and PGE_1 demonstrate stronger penile rigidity and higher success for PGE_1, but decreased penile pain and discomfort with moxisylyte.[49]

The improved understanding of smooth muscle physiology and agents producing relaxation has resulted in the development of K_{ATP} channel openers for the treatment of ED. These novel substances, which require intracavernosal injection, are being studied in early clinical trials with excellent, predictable erections without penile pain.[50] Recent clinical studies have confirmed the usefulness of injection therapy in the era of oral medications. Shabsigh *et al.*[51] demonstrated that alprostadil was effective, well tolerated and had a high satisfaction rate in salvaging men who had poor response to sildenafil. Mydlo *et al.*[52] have reported salvage using a combination of agents including sildenafil and alprostadil in men who do not have adequate responses to one agent alone.

While many men have been treated for many years for ED with intracavernosal injection therapy, there are complications and caveats regarding this form of therapy. Initial patient treatment and education should take place in the physician's office under controlled conditions. Patients should be given written information to take home about the technique of injection and possible side-effects. An initial, conservative dose should be tried and the patient observed for 30–60 minutes to be sure that a prolonged erection does not occur. Prolonged erections, defined as a rigid erection for more than 4 hours, should be treated with aspiration of the corpora and injection of an alpha stimulator such as phenylephrine in dilute concentration. Patients taking chronic injection therapy should be examined every 6–12 months for corporal fibrosis. While rare, corporal fibrosis may require change to a different agent, anti-inflammatory medications, or cessation of injection therapy.

Overall, this technique is simple and relatively painless to administer, effective and safe. Men need to be taught the technique carefully.

In the UK, alprostadil is available either in packs with syringes, needles and separate vials of powder and diluent for mixing (Caverject or Viridal) or with a simple injector

1. Remove an injection device and needle from the box. Peel the foil cover from the needle. Attach by pushing onto the tip of the device. Turn clockwise until it is firmly in place. Pull off the outer protective cap of the needle.

2. Hold the device with the needle pointing upwards. The white plunger rod is in the extended position.

3. Turn the plunger rod clockwise until it stops. This mixes the powder and diluent. Gently shake to make sure that the solution is evenly mixed. Do not use if it is cloudy or contains particles.

4. Hold the device with the needle upwards. Carefully remove the inner cap from the needle.

5. To remove any large bubbles, flick the cartridge with your finger, then keeping the device upright press the plunger rod as far as it will go. A few drops will appear at the needlepoint. It is normal for there to be small micro-bubbles at the side of the glass cartridge, which you can ignore.

6. Turn the end of the plunger rod slowly clockwise to select your dose. Your doctor will have told you what this should be. The number appearing in the window indicates the dose of the injection. If you make a mistake, continue to turn the plunger rod clockwise until you reach the correct dose.

7. Hold the penis between your thumb and forefinger as shown, and squeeze gently. The injection site will then bulge out. Make sure that the foreskin is stretched.

8. Push the needle all the way into the bulgy part ensuring that the syringe is held at a right angle (90 degrees) to the penis, avoiding obvious blood vessels.

9. Push the plunger firmly so that your dose is injected. Press gently on the needle mark and massage the penis to help the alprostdil to spread through. Dispose of the needle and syringe as recommended by your doctor or nurse.

You can prepare your injection up to 24 hours before using it provided it is kept at room temperature.

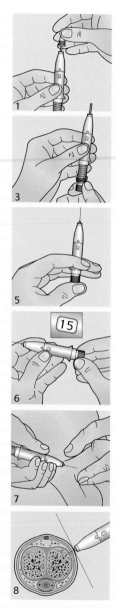

Figure 12a. Caverject Dual Chamber and instruction sheet.

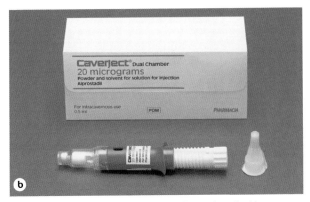

Figure 12b. Caverject Dual Chamber. Reproduced with permission from Pharmacia.

device, Caverject Dual Chamber (Figure 12a and b) or Viridal Duo (Figure 13). Currently, the Caverject Dual Chamber preparation is the easiest to use.

Most men will be suitable for injection treatment though caution should be exercised under certain circumstances (see Table 24).

Method of administration

Intracavernosal injection treatment involves the injection of a small volume (less than 1 ml) of the vasoactive drug

---

Table 24. Cautions regarding intracavernosal self-injection treatment for ED

Contraindications or caution should be exercised if:

- Haemoglobinopathy or bleeding diathesis
- Severe Peyronie's disease
- Poor manual dexterity
- Inadequate visual acuity
- Large abdomen, small penis preventing safe technique
- Needle-phobia or tendency to syncope
- Serious psychiatric disorders
- Likely abuse

into one of the corpora cavernosa. Men should be carefully instructed on its use to be sure they are going to be competent, safe and confident in its use.

Advice should be reinforced by written and pictorial instructions.

The foreskin should be retracted and the penis stretched by pulling (and at the same time protecting) the glans with one hand. The injection is then given into the top of the side of the shaft of the penis, avoiding any obvious superficial veins. Care should be taken to avoid the glans, the dorsal vein and the urethra ventrally.

An erection should occur in approximately 10 minutes and may last several hours. Excessive doses may produce a prolonged erection and priapism.

It is essential that this is explained and men given instructions on what action to take in such an event. An erection lasting more than 4 hours may require medical or surgical detumescence and men should be told to attend an emergency medicine department if this should occur. It is helpful if men have with them instructions for the emergency medical team in case they are unfamiliar with the problem (see Table 25).

Side-effects of intracavernosal injection treatment include:

- Bruising.
- Painful erection.
- Penile scarring.
- Infection (very rare).
- Prolonged erection if excessive dose.

Dosage should be determined by the man in his normal home environment rather than in a clinic/surgery. He should be given written instructions to start with a small dose and gradually increase on separate occasions until the lowest effective dose is found. Written instructions on incremental dose increases should be provided (see Table 26).

Intracavernosal injection treatment remains an important and effective treatment option, but is now usually second choice to oral treatments.

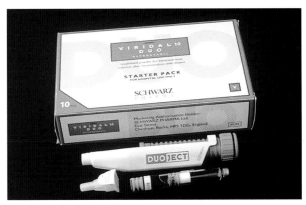

Figure 13. Viridal Duo. Reproduced with permission fromSchwarz Pharma

Table 25. Suggested treatment for prolonged erection

Erection still present 2–4 hours after injection:

Try local ice-packs

Try leg exercises – running, cycling

Erection still present >6 hours after injection:

Emergency hospital attendance mandatory for following procedure:

A 25-gauge butterfly needle is inserted into one corpora

Aspirate 50 ml of blood and apply pressure for 5 minutes

Aspirate a further 50 ml if the above fails, irrigate with heparinized saline and apply pressure

If this fails, then inject 200 micrograms of phenylephrine and repeat if necessary

If all measures fail, surgical treatment will be required

Table 26. Recommended doses for intracavernosal injection of vasoactive drugs

Alprostadil	Starting dose 5–10 mcg

	Incremental increases by
	        5 mcg up to 20 mcg
	        10 mcg up to 40 mcg

	Consider drug combinations if >40 mcg required
Papaverine	Starting dose 10 mg

	Incremental increases by
	        5 mg up to 20 mg
	        10 mg up to 60 mg

Combinations should start with combinations of minimum doses and increase by similar increments to those above. Phentolamine and VIP may be included in combinations.

Vacuum tumescence devices (VTDs)

Vacuum pumps for the treatment of ED have been around for many years. The design was first patented in 1917 by Otto Lederer. The basic principle remains unchanged, but there are now a variety of designs available (Figure 13). VTDs consist of a cylinder and vacuum pump to produce an erection and a constriction ring to maintain it .

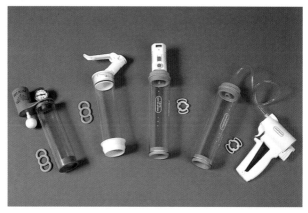

Figure 14. Vacuum devices.

Table 27. Categories of patient entitled to free NHS prescriptions for treatment of ED in the UK (prescriptions should be endorsed SLS*)

Those having diabetes, multiple sclerosis, Parkinson's disease, poliomyelitis, prostate cancer, severe pelvic injury, single gene neurological disorder, spina bifida or spinal cord injury

Those receiving dialysis for renal failure

Those that have had radical pelvic surgery, prostatectomy or kidney transplant

Those receiving ED treatment on 14 September 1998

Those suffering severe distress as a result of impotence (prescribed by specialist centre)

*selected list scheme

The erection produced is not physiologically normal. The penis becomes engorged and distended distal to the constricting ring, but will tend to pivot proximal to the ring. The penis will appear rather cyanosed and cold and may become painful with time. The ring should not be left on for more than 30 minutes.

VTDs are effective in approximately 70–80% of users, but this is dependent upon patient acceptability.[53] Couples with a good and open general and sexual relationship are most likely to be suitable for this form of therapy, and long-term usage appears to be as good if not better than self-injection therapy. Others may find them rather intrusive and contrived.

VTDs may also appear expensive, involving a capital outlay of £90–300 depending upon the type. In the long term, this is cost effective compared with oral or self-injection therapy. VTDs are now, like other treatments, available on a National Health Service free prescription in the UK for certain categories of patient (see Table 27).

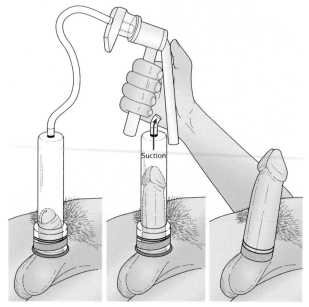

Figure 15. Schematic representation of use of a vacuum device.

Method of use of VTDs (see Figure 15)
- It is helpful to obtain a video instruction with the device.
- The device needs to be used in conjunction with sexual arousal.
- Devices consist of a plastic cylinder, a vacuum pump and a constriction ring.
- Lubricant is applied to the penis and inside the cylinder.
- The constriction ring is placed around the base of the cylinder.
- The cylinder with attached or integral vacuum pump is placed over the penis and pressed firmly against the body to produce an air-tight seal.
- The vacuum pump is operated and continued until adequate tumescence is produced.

- The constriction ring is then slipped off the cylinder base and onto the base of the penis.
- The cylinder is then removed.
- The ring is carefully removed after sexual activity. It should never be left on for more than 30 minutes.

Vacuum devices are usually used alone, but can be used in conjunction with other treatments to augment the effect.

Complications and disadvantages of VTDs include:

- Haematoma or petechiae.
- Coldness of penis.
- Pivoting of penile base.
- Ejaculatory block.
- Discomfort.
- Cumbersome and unnatural.

Relative contraindications of VTDs include:

- Poor manual dexterity.
- Bleeding diatheses.
- Sickle cell trait or disease.
- Anticoagulant treatments.

There is now available a wide selection of devices, and some types and addresses are shown in Appendix 3.

Vacuum devices can be a very effective treatment for men with ED, but do require careful selection and care to use the device properly. Most studies have shown reasonable patient and partner satisfaction.[54]

Most companies will provide a helpline for advice for men who have initial difficulty using the device. Most companies will also include a "money back if not satisfied" clause provided the device is returned within a designated period of time.

The choice of device will depend upon availability, price and personal preference.

Surgical treatment

Surgical treatment of ED is considered third-line therapy and is used in men when more conservative therapy is contraindicated or ineffective. The majority of these men suffer from significant vascular disease, penile corpus cavernosum fibrosis from priapism, have anatomical abnormalities such as Peyronie's disease or through choice prefer surgery to correct their ED. Options for the surgical treatment of ED include implantation of penile prosthesis, penile vein ligation for venous incompetence, or vascular bypass surgery for arterial abnormalities. The last two options are rarely used even in an ED referral practice. While surgical intervention may be more reliable in certain selected patients, the incidence of morbidity and complications are significantly greater than medical treatment.

Penile prosthesis implants

Prosthetic implants to restore erectile function have been attempted for many years. Early prosthetic implants using rib cartilage, acrylic implanted beneath Buck's fascia and other plastic devices were poorly tolerated, resulted in inadequate erectile function, and frequently resulted in infection, extrusion and pain. Rehabilitation for ED with these devices was never successful.[55] The development of newer synthetic materials in the 1950s and 1960s allowed improved prosthetic design, greater acceptance and satisfaction. The silicone-based prosthetic materials introduced as a result of the space programme furthered the science of human prosthetics and penile prosthetic devices. The development of silicone elastomer has revolutionized these prostheses and provided a material which is durable, easily fashioned into useful urological prosthetic devices, associated with minimal infection, and excellent tissue compatibility.

Initial silicone penile prostheses were introduced for implantation within the corpora cavernosa by Small et al.[56] and Scott et al.,[57] who introduced semi-rigid rod and inflatable penile prostheses, respectively. These two early reports define the two current classes of penile prostheses that are most commonly implanted today. Current prosthetic devices include the inflatable variety, which can be divided into multiple component inflatable penile prostheses, of which there are two- and three-piece models. Semi-rigid rod prostheses continue to be available and grouped as malleable prostheses that contain a central metal wire for improved positioning and mechanical prostheses such as the Dura II penile prosthesis. The design of these devices and their surgical implantation have been widely reported and are clearly documented.[55,58]

All of these implantable devices are sized at the time of surgery, provide excellent penile rigidity and size, and simulate normal physiological erections adequate for sexual intercourse. The flaccid state differs with the type of device selected.

Semi-rigid rod penile prostheses

The semi-rigid rod penile prostheses were the first prostheses designed for restoration of erections and erectile function (Figure 16). A variety of semi-rigid rod penile prostheses of different designs are currently available. These devices, which are most extensively used, consist of two full, but flexible, rods or cylinders which can be varied in length by trimming the proximal portion or adding measured extensions to the proximal portion to fit the individual patient's measurements. Designs usually include a central braided metal wire, allowing for positioning of the prosthesis when not in use. Mechanical modifications of these devices include hinges increasing the flexibility and positioning ability of the prosthesis.

Surgical implantation of these prostheses is the simplest of penile prosthesis implantations. A subcoronal, dorsal penile, ventral penile or perineal incision may be used to access the corpora cavernosa for implantation. Once Buck's fascia has been dissected away from the tunica albuginea, a corporotomy incision is carried out through the tunica albuginea to reveal the underlying corpus cavernosum tissue. This tissue is then dilated with Hegar or Brooks dilators of 8–13 mm diameter. The length of

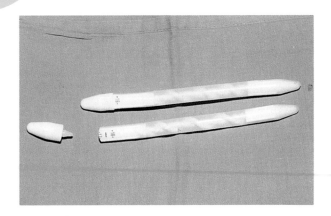

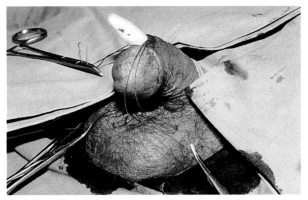

Figure 16. Semi-rigid prosthetic insertion. Reproduced with permission from Eardley I, Sethia K. *Erectile Dysfunction: Current Investigation and Management*. London: Mosby, 2003.

the corpora cavernosa from just proximal to the glans penis to the crura of the corpora cavernosa is measured using a metal sizer. Once measured, the appropriate penile prosthesis length is obtained and inserted. Care must be taken to seat the prosthesis both proximal and distally, such that migration is unlikely to occur. Excessive length may preclude accurate positioning, promote cylinder extrusion or produce distal penile pain. The tunica albuginea incisions are closed with absorbable or non-absorbable sutures. Patients can begin use of their implant at 4–6 weeks following surgery.

Inflatable penile prostheses

Inflatable penile prostheses are available in self-contained, two-piece and three-piece designs (see Figure 17). Self-contained penile prostheses are modifications of semi-rigid and inflatable prostheses in which each cylinder contains an inflation chamber, pump and proximal reservoir. The device is inflated by pressure on the distal portion of each cylinder just proximal to the glans penis. This pressure fills each cylinder with fluid supplied from the proximal reservoir. While little distension of these cylinders occurs, rigidity can be expected from appropriate inflation. Deflation is carried out by exerting external pressure on the cylinders by deflecting them inferiorly. A release valve in the pump mechanism produces return of fluid from the inflatable portion of the prosthesis to the reservoir with increased pressure. These prostheses are implanted like semi-rigid rod prostheses.

Two-piece inflatable penile prostheses are designed to contain two completely inflatable cylinders and a pump/reservoir placed in the scrotum. This pump/reservoir provides limited but usually adequate fluid volume for inflation and deflation of the prosthesis. The two-piece design avoids abdominal placement of a fluid reservoir used in the three-piece inflatable prostheses. The two-piece design has an advantage over the self-contained prostheses in that it increases the volume of fluid placed in the penile cylinders to improve both erectile inflation and flaccidity between uses. Because of pump/reservoir volume, however, flaccidity may not be as complete as with three-piece inflatable prostheses. Implantation of these devices is similar to that described below for the three-piece inflatable penile prosthesis.

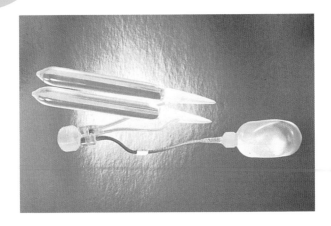

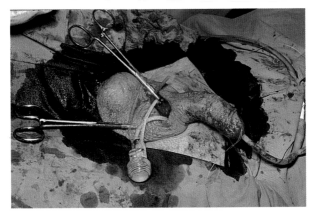

Figure 17. Inflatable prosthetic insertion. Reproduced with permission from Eardley I, Sethia K. *Erectile Dysfunction: Current Investigation and Management*. London: Mosby, 2003.

Three-piece inflatable penile prostheses are the most complex, yet the most satisfactory, physiological prosthetic devices available. This prosthesis consists of two inflatable hollow cylinders placed in the corpora cavernosa and connected to a small pump device used to inflate and deflate the prosthesis, which is placed in the scrotum lateral to the testicle. Fluid is provided by a fluid reservoir placed beneath the rectus muscles of the abdomen. Because of the significant volume of fluid in this reservoir for both inflation and deflation, the erect and flaccid states are generally excellent. These devices provide increased girth and length in comparison to other devices. Similarly, the improved flaccidity facilitates positioning and carriage of the prosthesis under clothing and overall cosmetic appearance.

Surgical procedure

Inflatable penile prostheses may be placed through an infrapubic or penoscrotal approach. Following incision, the corpora cavernosa are exposed bilaterally, as described previously. If approached dorsally, the neurovascular bundle between the corpora cavernosa is carefully protected and the urethra carefully protected with the penoscrotal incision. Once the corpora cavernosa are identified, Buck's fascia is dissected away from the tunica albuginea and the tunica albuginea opened. Dissection into the corpora cavernosa through the corporotomy incision is carried out with scissors and Hager or Brooks dilators, as described previously. Gentle dilation of each corpus cavernosum is then performed from the distal-most portion of the distal corpus cavernosum just proximal to the glans penis to the crura of the corpora cavernosa at their attachments to the pubic bone. Dilation is carried out from 8 to 13 mm, followed by careful size measurement of each corpus cavernosum using the Furlow or Jonas sizing tool. Cylinders are chosen after sizing and additional length is added by rear tip extenders until the cylinder size and the previously measured size are equivalent. The prostheses are positioned in each corpus cavernosum using the Furlow insertion tool.

A pouch is then created beneath the rectus muscle for the reservoir for three-piece prostheses and in the scrotum lateral to the testicle for both the two-piece and the three-piece prostheses. These pouches are created using sharp and blunt dissection. The incision is then closed using absorbable or non-absorbable sutures. The reservoir is placed beneath the rectus muscle and the pump in the scrotal pouch. Once all components of the prosthesis are placed, the reservoir is filled and tubing connected if preconnected devices are not used. The device is inflated and deflated to evaluate penile shape, position, size, and adequacy of erection and flaccidity. Thorough irrigation with antibiotic solution and preoperative intravenous antibiotic administration are recommended. A suction drain and Foley catheter may be placed at the surgeon's discretion.

Postoperative care

Postoperatively, patients are covered with additional antibiotics, an ice pack is applied to the genitalia and patients are asked to check pump positioning for at least 4 weeks before activation of inflatable devices. Oral analgesics are administered. Patients are then asked to return for device activation 2–6 weeks postoperatively.

Peyronie's disease

Penile prostheses have frequently been used for the treatment of patients with ED associated with significant Peyronie's disease with or without penile curvature.[55] Many patients do not respond to penile straightening alone because of inadequate erectile function, severe penile curvature or significant penile shortening; penile prostheses have been used successfully to rehabilitate these complex patients with significant ED. In counselling patients about surgical treatment of severe Peyronie's disease, it is important to include the option of penile prosthesis, since this single surgical procedure has excellent success, low morbidity, and corrects both penile deformity and potential ED. Excellent results have been reported by many investigators using penile prosthesis implantation with and without corpus cavernosum reconstruction.[58]

While corpus cavernosum reconstruction is occasionally required to produce penile straightening, the recent introduction of penile modelling has reduced the number of incisions, the use of additional foreign bodies for penile straightening and reduced postoperative morbidity in patients with significant penile curvature. The inflatable penile prosthesis has been demonstrated to have the best long-term patient satisfaction in the treatment of patients with penile curvature and Peyronie's disease.[59]

Corpus cavernosum fibrosis and priapism

Dense fibrosis of the corpus cavernosum can result from a variety of conditions, including repeated intracorporal injections, cavernositis following penile prosthesis infection, diabetes mellitus, Peyronie's disease, and most often, priapism. This fibrosis, whether mild or severe, results in abnormal corpus cavernosum tissue compliance with an increased incidence of venous leak and decreased penile turgidity. Penile prosthesis is the most common successful method for rehabilitating patients with these disabling conditions. When attempting penile prosthesis placement in these difficult clinical conditions, it is critical to have available downsized inflatable penile prosthesis cylinders available. These devices are available from both Mentor and American Medical Systems as the AMS 700CXM and permit placement of a prosthesis in a seriously fibrotic corpus cavernosum.

A vacuum erection device can be used preoperatively to increase penile length, and assist in softening corporal fibrosis in men with severe corpus cavernosum fibrosis and scarring. Patients are asked to apply the device two to three times weekly without a constriction ring for 8–12 weeks. Use of a vacuum device with an implanted, functioning penile prosthesis has been reported, but may result in damage to a functioning, implanted device. If all dilation attempts are unsuccessful, a longitudinal incision in the corpus cavernosum can be carried out with dissection of the fibrotic tissue from the corpus cavernosum. This is a difficult procedure and requires significant care to avoid the urethra and other penile structures. Once performed, however, a prosthetic cylinder may be placed in the open dissected area and covered with tunica albuginea, autologous or synthetic graft material.[59] If inflation of the prosthesis is unsuccessful, the use of a semi-rigid rod device may be necessary to permit satisfactory prosthesis function. Penile implants have been successfully implanted in patients with sickle cell priapism with excellent results.

Penile prosthesis implantation following radical prostatectomy

Despite the advent of nerve-sparing radical prostatectomy, as many as 60% of men undergoing radical prostatectomy will suffer ED. While many of these men can be satisfactorily managed with oral, intraurethral or injectable agents, some patients will require penile prosthesis implantation. In patients with preoperatively placed penile prosthesis, there is no clear indication for removal of a pre-existing penile prosthesis during or before radical retropubic prostatectomy. Others have suggested the immediate and simultaneous placement of penile prosthesis along with radical prostatectomy. Similarly, patients have excellent function and penile prosthesis satisfaction following definitive radiation therapy for prostatic carcinoma.

Penile prosthesis and spinal cord injury

Patients suffering from spinal cord injury may also require penile prosthesis implantation. Results of these procedures in patients with spinal cord injury will assist in rehabilitation, especially in patients who are not responsive to less invasive methods for restoring erectile function.[59]

Paraplegic men may benefit from a semi-rigid rod prosthesis, as these devices can produce good erections and at the same time facilitate adherence of condom catheter urinary collection systems.

Penile reconstruction

One of the most difficult groups of patients to treat are those patients with penile loss secondary to congenital absence, trauma avulsion or penectomy for carcinoma of the penis. A variety of phallic reconstruction techniques are available. The most commonly used procedure is an innervated vascularized pedicle flap from the forearm. Following phallic reconstruction, penile prosthesis implantation permits a functional penis.[59] Reconstruction with a neourethra allows for normal voiding and penile prostheses permit sexual activity. Because these phallic reconstructive techniques involve nerve reconstruction, sensation can be expected in the majority of patients. Inflatable and semi-rigid rod penile prostheses following these phallic reconstructions can restore the ability to have adequate coitus. Similarly, the self-contained penile prosthesis has been used successfully in reconstructions for female to male transsexuals.

Postoperative complications

Although postoperative complications have decreased markedly in the past decade, mechanical malfunction may still occur with any of the penile prosthetic devices. Semi-rigid rod penile prostheses can sustain cable fracture and decreased rigidity over time and require replacement. Inflatable prostheses, however, are more likely to sustain mechanical complications. Reported mechanical malfunctions and malfunction rates are currently below 5% for 3 years with fluid leak continuing to be the most common problem with inflatable penile prostheses. These fluid leaks are most commonly located in the cylinders, which are the highest pressure portion of the device. Device malfunction requires surgical exploration, with replacement of device portions which have malfunctioned.

Additional complications include infection, which occurs in less than 5% of patients with penile prostheses. Higher infection rates can be expected in patients with prosthesis revisions, autoimmune diseases and diabetes mellitus. Newer design penile prostheses have included antibiotic-coated devices to reduce infection. These recently developed implants are coated with a combination of rifampin and minocycline, and have been reported to have a more than 60% reduction of infection rates. With this combination of antibiotics, the most common pathogens, *Staphyloccus aureus* and *Staphylococcus epidermidis*, are rarely encountered. Prosthesis removal, healing and later replacement constitutes the conservative method for patients with penile prosthesis infections.

Most patients now have a salvage procedure[60] where the infected implant is removed, the wound is irrigated with multiple antibiotic solutions and a new sterile prosthesis is implanted in the same operation. The advantages of this latter approach are the preservation of penile size, length and sensation, with few recurrant infections. Additional complications include prosthesis erosion, prolonged pain, and decreased penile sensation and length. These complications, while rare, are of significant concern to the implanting surgeon.

Patient and partner satisfaction

A number of studies have investigated surgical success and degree of postoperative satisfaction in patients undergoing penile prosthesis implantation. The success of surgical outcome is associated with patient and partner relationship concerns and the patient's preoperative psychological status.

One study comparing satisfaction rates with the two types of prostheses identified no significant difference in satisfaction by the patient with the two types of prostheses, but an increased satisfaction with inflatable implants when the patient's sexual partner was surveyed. Satisfaction rates, however, are high for all types of implanted penile prostheses.[58,61,62]

Surgery for veno-occlusive incompetence

Surgical procedures for venous incompetence or venous leak ED are designed to increase venous outflow resistance from the sinusoidal spaces of the corpora cavernosa. Patients are evaluated prior to these surgical procedures with radiographic studies called cavernosography and cavernosometry. Studies begin with intracavernosal injection of alprostadil or papavarine to stimulate an erection. Blood flow is measured by pulsed Doppler flow ultrasonography The use of these diagnostic procedures following injection of vasoactive agents will accurately identify patients with ED as a result of venous leakage or incompetence. These patients with veno-occlusive dysfunction typically complain of firm erections for short periods of time, described as partial and fleeting. Their erections are difficult to maintain. These men are typically in their twenties to forties and often report primary ED with no erections as adolescents or young adults.[63] Patients may be candidates for surgery for venous incompetence if studies of arterial inflow demonstrate normal arterial blood flow. Patients thus selected are candidates for crural plication, deep penile dorsal vein excision and ligation, or dorsal vein arterialization.

Surgical procedure

After placement of a Foley catheter for urethral identification, a curvilinear inguinal scrotal incision is carried out lateral to the base of the penis. The corpus cavernosum crus is exposed along its attachment to the ischiopubic ramus. Multiple plication sutures are applied to the ventral aspect of the crura to decrease venous outflow from the crura of the corpora cavernosa.

The penis is then dissected free and identified from the suspensory ligament to the glans penis by inverting the penis from its skin. The deep dorsal vein is identified beneath Buck's fascia and ligated from an area proximal to the suspensory ligament to the distal pendulous penis. The deep dorsal vein is excised with multiple ligations of the cavernosal veins along the extent of the dorsal vein. In proximal ligation, care must be taken to avoid the carvernosal nerve and the dorsal nerves of the penis must be avoided during deep dorsal vein excision. At the conclusion of the procedure, a suction drain is placed subcutaneously and the incision closed. The patients are treated with ice packs and oral analgesics postoperatively.

While many patients sustain venous incompetence as a cause of their ED, the results of surgical intervention have been poor. Surgical success has been achieved in less than 40% of patients, with an additional 40% responding to a combination of surgery and vasoactive injectable agents.[64] Complications include penile shortening, decreased penile sensation, recurrent venous incompetence and wound infection. Because of the variable success of these procedures, venous ligation procedures should only be performed in highly selected patients who are acutely aware of possible failures and outcomes.

Arterial revascularization

Highly selected patients with arterial lesions, usually traumatically acquired and without significant atherosclerosis or atherosclerotic risk factors, may be selected for penile arterial revascularization or deep dorsal vein arterialization. Since high blood flow rates produce erectile function in the corpora cavernosa, the integrity of arterial supply is critical for normal erectile function.[65] Once pulsed Doppler ultrasound with intracavernosal injection diagnostic studies have demonstrated reduced arterial blood flow abnormalities, arteriography after the stimulation of the corpus cavernosum with vasoactive agents will document arterial abnormalities in the internal iliac and pudendal arteries. Specific arteriographic visualization of the internal pudendal arteries and central cavernosal arteries is essential for the diagnosis of arterial compromise in these patients. In patients selected for surgical procedures, alternatives of surgical intervention must be discussed, including the possibility of penile prosthesis implantation. Appropriate candidates are usually less than 40 years of age, non-smokers, with normal cholesterol, and with single arterial lesions of traumatic aetiology.

Surgical procedures

In lesions which are unlikely to respond to percutaneous transluminal angioplasty, arterial revascularization may be considered. A variety of procedures have been designed for arterial revascularization. Each of these depends upon the use of the inferior epigastric artery, which is dissected free from the underside of the rectus muscle and rooted to the penile vasculature. Since the central cavernosal arteries are relatively inaccessible to revascularization, the deep dorsal artery is a better choice for anastomosis of the inferior epigastric artery. This can be performed in an end-to-end or end-to-side fashion, with distal ligation of the dorsal artery of the penis to redirect blood to the central cavernosal arteries.

An incision is carried out lateral to the rectus muscle and the entire length of the inferior epigastric artery unilaterally or bilaterally is exposed through the rectus sheath. The vessel is then re-routed to pass deep to the rectus muscle. The inferior epigastric artery is mobilized with its communicating veins and after tunnelling above the pubic bone, the inferior epigastric artery is placed at the proximal distal portion of the penis. A transverse or longitudinal incision is then carried out near the base of the penis to expose at least one of the dorsal penile arteries or veins for anastomosis. An end-to-end or end-to-side anastomosis is carried out using microscopic surgical techniques after removal of ellipses of the vascular wall of the recipient vessel. A 2-mm anastomosis is carried out using 10-0 nylon suture. Following release of vascular clamps, blood flow is easily identified in all limbs of the anastomosis with excellent postoperative blood flow.

While complications from this procedure are few, excessive arterial blood flow may result in priapism or glans penis hyperaemia. Similarly, the anastomosis may occlude during the follow-up. Patients are encouraged to avoid sexual activity for approximately 6 weeks postoperatively. While the results of these procedures vary widely with the reported surgical experiences, as many as 65% of patients have reported return of coitus following arterial bypass grafts.[64,66] With careful selection of patients, careful surgical technique and long term follow-up, outcomes will continue to improve.

Priapism: Aetiology, Diagnosis and Treatment

Priapism is named after Priapus, the Greek god of fertility. Priapism is an abnormal penile erection which is generally not initiated by sexual stimulation. Priapism is an urgent medical condition that requires evaluation and often rapid treatment to avoid loss of erectile function. This condition is most common in men but has been reported in women as clitoral priapism. It usually involves the paired corpora cavernosa with a rigid penile shaft with flaccid glans penis and corpus spongiosum. Rare cases involve the corpus spongiosum. Stuttering priapism is defined as recurrent, intermittent, painful erections. Priapism associated with haematological or solid malignant disease is a rare condition. Metastasis of solid tumours to the penis, including bladder (32%) and prostate (28%), are the most common, followed by kidney (17%), gastrointestinal (8%), and rarely from testis, lung, liver, bone and sarcomas.[66] While the mechanism of malignant priapism remains controversial, this condition may be due to penile tissue replacement by malignant tissue, venous obstruction, or abnormal stimulus of the afferent or efferent neural pathways stimiulating erection.[67]

Incidence

A population-based retrospective cohort study found an overall incidence rate of 1.5 per 100,000 person-years, while the incidence rate in men 40 years old and older was 2.9 per 100,000 person-years.[68] In patients using intracorporal injection therapy for erectile dysfunction (ED), priapism or prolonged erection may be seen in 1% of men taking PGE_1 and in up to 17% of those on papaverine injection.[69] Priapism is quite common in patients with sickle cell trait and disease. Self-limited priapistic episodes, usually during sleep, occur commonly and last less than 3 hours. Priapism associated with sickle cell anaemia (SCA) is unusual before puberty and occurs in approximately 6% of children with SCA. No correlations are observed between the frequency of priapic episodes and episode duration. A study of SCA men after puberty reported a prevalence of priapism of 42%.[70] Priapism in that study was associated with low haemoglobin F and high platelet counts. More than 25% of men who had priapism had some degree of ED. In patients with homozygous SCA and sickle cell beta(0) thalassaemia between 5 and 20 years of age, there is an 89% probability of priapism by age 20, with the mean duration of an episode of approximately 125 minutes. These episodes usually occur around 4 a.m., and 75% of the patients have at least one episode starting during sleep or at awakening.[70]

Other risk factors for priapism include cocaine drug use, advanced pelvic or haematological malignancy, amyloidosis, and those on warfarin, heparin and certain antipsychotic drugs.[71,72] Other uncommon aetiologies include glucose phosphate isomerase deficiency and Fabry's disease, and total parenteral nutrition treatment with especially high doses of androgens has been associated with priapism in hypogonadal men receiving gonadotropin-releasing hormone or high-dose testosterone.[73,74] Testosterone-induced priapism in adolescents with SCA, and priapism after androstenedione intake for athletic performance enhancement, have been reported.[75–77] Table 28 lists the aetiologies of ischaemic priapism as reported by the American Foundation for Urologic Disease (AFUD) Panel on Priapism[66] and Table 29 shows the aetiological factors in priapism.[78]

The AFUD panel on priapism outlined an algorithm for the definition and treatment of priapism. They defined ischaemic priapism (veno-occlusive), the most common form of priapism, as a painful, rigid erection characterized by absent cavernous arterial or venous blood flow. Ischaemic priapism of 4 hours or more duration is a "compartment syndrome" requiring emergency medical

Table 28. Aetiology of priapism (AFUD classification)
Drug-induced
Haematological
Sickle cell disease and other haemoglobinopathies
Thrombophilia states (protein C and other thrombophilias, lupus)
Hyperviscosity states (hyperleukocytosis, polycythaemia)
Idiopathic
CNS mediated
Other

intervention. Potential sequelae are irreversible corporal fibrosis and permanent ED.

The combination of venous outflow obstruction, high-pressure chambers and poor-to-absent inflow can lead to trabecular interstitial oedema and ultrastructural changes in trabecular smooth muscle cells and functional transformation to fibroblast-like cells. In priapism lasting more than 24 hours, severe cellular damage and widespread necrosis may occur.[78] Destruction of the endothelial lining, formation of blood clots within the corpora and widespread transformation of the smooth muscle cells to fibroblast-like cells or necrosis occurs in cases lasting beyond 48 hours and eventually results in irreversible ED.[78] Lack of these changes in priapism lasting less than 12 hours emphasizes the importance of patient education and early intervention.

In an animal model, anoxia has been shown to eliminate spontaneous and drug-induced contractile activity, suggesting a likely explanation for the failure of penile injection of alpha-adrenergic agonists to reverse prolonged ischaemic priapism when the penis is in its maximal rigid state.[79] The failure of detumescence seen in low-flow priapism may be secondary to failed alpha-adrenergic neurotransmission, endothelin deficit or inactivation of intracellular cofactors of smooth muscle contraction due to hypoxia and /or hypercarbia.[79]

Table 29. Aetiological factors in priapism

Low-flow states (veno-occlusive or ischaemic type)

Haemoglobinopathies and sickle cell disease

Thrombophilia states (lupus, protein C)

Warfarin/heparin-induced

Fabry's disease

Dialysis

TPN (high fat content)

Vasculitis

Haematological malignancies

Pelvic/lower GU tract (bladder and prostate) cancer and metastatic (i.e. renal) malignancies

Psychotropics and antidepressants (chlorpromazine, trazodone, risperidol)

Antihypertensives (guanethidine, hydralazine, prazosin)

Erectogenic agents (intracavernosal vasoactives, sildenafil, intraurethral PGE1)

Spinal cord stenosis

Amyloidosis

Glucose phosphate isomerase deficiency

Alcohol

Androgens/testosterone

High-flow states (arterial or non-ischaemic type)

Penile/perineal trauma

- Straddle injury

- Cavernosal artery injury

- Arteriosinusoidal fistula

Cocaine

Metastatic malignancy

Fabry's disease

Iatrogenic (following deep dorsal vein arterialization)

From a neurological standpoint, the efferent erectile pathway is via the pelvic nerves, which are joined by the preganglionic parasympathetic nerves. The pelvic nerves join the pelvic plexus, which gives rise to the cavernous nerve of the penis. Normally, penile stimulation will cause reflexogenic erections that are primarily controlled by the sacral parasympathetic nerves originating from the S2–S4 segment located at the T11–L1 vertebral levels. The afferent limb of the erection response is mediated by the dorsal penile nerve (a branch of the pudendal nerve), which transmits sensory impulses to the spinal cord. The role of the sympathetic nervous system in penile erection is not entirely clear, but its activation is generally associated with contraction of corpus cavernosal smooth muscle and penile detumescence. The neuropathophysiology of priapism in patients with lumbar stenosis has not been fully elucidated, but it is postulated that it may be due to parasympathetic efferent hyperactivity in the S2–S4 cauda equina nerve roots within the narrowed thecal sac. The parasympathetic hyperactivity may be secondary to increased intrathecal pressure at the stenotic level and altered circulation within the cauda equina during walking.[79]

Drug-induced priapism has been reported with a variety of medications, most commonly related to the antihypertensive drugs guanethidine, prazosin and hydralazine, as well as psychotropic medications.[79] Antipsychotics are associated with a small, but definite, risk of priapism and the most commonly cited agents are trazodone (desyrel), thioridazine and chlorpromazine.[79] Psychotropic-induced priapism is almost always associated with low-flow pathology and is currently believed to be caused by the alpha-1-adrenergic antagonism of these medications. Chlorpromazine and thioridazine are conventional antipsychotics with the greatest alpha-1-adrenergic affinity and have been most frequently reported to be associated with priapism.[71] The exact pathophysiology has not been elucidated, but is likely multifactorial and may be related to the ratio of alpha-adrenergic blockade to anticholinergic activity. Risperidone, olanzapine and clozapine are the atypical antipsychotics that have been reported to cause priapism on rare occasions.[70]

Sickle cell haemoglobinopathy results from the inheritance of one or two genes coding for an abnormal S haemoglobin and manifests in 0.15% of black Americans in the form of sickle cell disease (homozygous for haemoglobin S) and in 8% as sickle cell trait (heterozygous for haemoglobin S). Inheritance of a combination of a haemoglobin S gene and a second gene coding for an abnormal haemoglobin (i.e. B[+] thalassaemia or C haemoglobin) is possible and, as in the homozygous type, may result in ischaemic complications.[69] The pathophysiology of SCA-induced priapism is thought to result from decreased oxygen tension and pH developing in stagnant blood within the corporal sinusoids, which in turn leads to a cycle of erythrocyte sickling and sludging, followed by even more hypoxaemia and acidosis.[80]

High-flow, non-ischaemic or arterial priapism is a less common form of priapism that presents clinically as a painless erection that typically follows some type of penile or perineal trauma leading to unregulated arterial inflow into the sinusoidal space. The following represents the AFUD panel[66] agreement on classification of non-ischaemic priapism:

Non-ischaemic (arterial) priapism is a less common form of priapism caused by unregulated cavernous inflow.

The erection is usually painless and not fully rigid.

Non-ischaemic priapism requires evaluation but is not a compartment syndrome nor a medical emergency.

Different from veno-occlusive, high-flow priapism is not an emergency: the penile venous outflow mechanism remains intact and the cavernosal tissue remains well oxygenated. The penis is not usually rigid in these men and intercourse may be possible. The onset of priapism following perineal trauma is often delayed and may consist of persistent partial rigidity with increased rigidity on arousal.[80] Diagnosis is based on clinical history, physical examination and a demonstration of arterial blood on aspirated cavernosal blood gas measurements. Investigators have shown that, at the level of trabecular smooth muscle cells, the ultrastructural changes and fibroblast-like cellular transformation seen in low-flow states do not occur with high-flow priapism, with long duration.[79] The pathophysiology of high-flow priapism is not like that of an arteriovenous fistula; the condition can be defined as an arterial lacunar fistula, where the helicine arteries and their control mechanisms are bypassed and the blood passes directly into the lacunar spaces. The high flow in the lacunar space creates shear stress, leading to increased NO release, activation of the cGMP pathway and smooth muscle relaxation, with resultant trabecular dilatation.[80] The delay in the onset of high-flow priapism may be caused by a delay in the destruction of the arterial wall after the initial penile/perineal trauma. Alternatively, the delay may be secondary to clot formation at the site of injury, followed by the normal lytic pathways and an opening of the fistulous tract.

Diagnosis and treatment

The physician must initially distinguish arterial from venoocclusive priapism. The AFUD panel algorithm for the treatment of priapism is outlined in Figure 18.[66,81] A complete medical history and physical examination are the cornerstones of accurate diagnosis and effective treatment. The history should include medications, trauma and predisposing risk factors. Severity of pain is a fairly reliable predictor of low-flow priapism. High-flow priapism is suggested by penile or perineal trauma. Absence of pain in high-flow priapism frequently results in less pain and associated patient anxiety than veno-occlusive priapism. Physical examination is essential and will reveal firm corpora cavernosa and a soft, flaccid glans penis and corpus spongiosum. Laboratory studies should include screening for psychoactive drugs and metabolites of cocaine.[72] The AFUD panel has recommended reticulocyte count, urinalysis, CBC, platelets and differential white blood count.

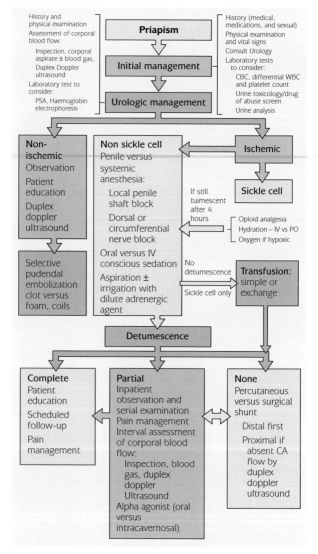

Figure 18. Treatment model for management of priapism. Reproduced with permission from Berger R *et al*. Report of the American Foundation for Urologic Disease (AFUD) Thought Leader Panel for evaluation and treatment of priapism. *Int J Impotence Res* 2001; **13**(Suppl 5): S39–S43.[66]

Urological management after these basic measures includes assessment of corporal blood flow status with corporal aspirate and visual inspection by blood colour and consistency. Corporal blood gas including pH, PO_2 and PCO_2 will quantitate these findings or a penile duplex Doppler ultrasound will show compromised blood flow. Low-flow priapism is suggested by low oxygen tension, high carbon dioxide and low serum pH in the aspirate. When high-flow priapsim is suspected based on the bright red blood or blood gas analysis, duplex Doppler sonography may identify a dilated cavernosal artery or pseudocapsule formation at the site of arterial sinusoidal fistula. These findings will be helpful if superselective arterial embolization is necessary.[81] Since the management of the low-flow and high-flow states is radically different, sonography should be considered if conventional corporal irrigation and intracavernosal sympathomimetics (i.e. phenylephrine) fail to resolve the initial veno-occlusive priapism.[82] When a haemoglobinopathy is suspected, haemoglobin electrophoresis should be performed.

Treatment options must be selected based on priapism aetiology. For patients with non-sickle cell, low-flow priapism, initial pain control should include local penile block or regional/general anaesthesia in the form of dorsal nerve block, circumferential penile block, subcutaneous local penile shaft block, and oral or intravenous conscious sedation for the pediatric patient. The initial diagnostic penile aspiration is also used as initiation of therapy and aspiration of blood should be combined with intra-cavernosal injection of a sympathomimetic agent such as phenylephrine to promote detumescence This injection may be contraindicated in patients with cardiac disease or labile hypertension. Significant increases in blood pressure are possible and vital sign monitoring is essential when using any sympathomimetic agent. Because of its potent and highly selective alpha-1-adrenergic stimulatory properties and lack of beta stimulatory effect, often responsible for arrhythmias and angina, phenylephrine is the best choice for producing detumescence. If the initial injection is not successful, irrigation with saline usually containing a dilute solutin of phenylepherine is added.

Most cases of veno-occlusive, low-flow priapism treated within 12 hours of onset will respond to alpha agonist therapy and resolve within 20 minutes of infusion of a 500 microgram/ml phenylephrine solution with an infused dose of less than 1 mg. The AFUD consensus panel recommended first-line treatment of aspiration and irrigation for low-flow priapism of more than 4 hours duration before considering more invasive alternatives such as surgical shunts, since these surgical procedures have been associated with severe ED when priapism has persisted beyond 72 hours.[66]

Failure of resolution after conservative measures requires moving on to surgical intervention. A number of surgical shunts for diversion of blood out of the corpus cavernosum have been described. The most commonly used is the distal corporospongiosal shunt (Figure 19) and should be attempted before proximal shunts. The choice of percutaneous or open surgical shunt remains controversial. The simplest alternative is the transglanular Winter shunt (Figure 20), performed using a biopsy gun to create multiple channels between the corpus spongiosum and the corpora cavernosa.[83] If this technique is not successful, a larger communication between the corpora cavernosal and the corpus spongiosum may be created by an Al-Ghorab shunt, in which the distal tunica albuginea of the corpora cavernosa is removed through a transglanular incision. Proximal shunts have been reported and are recommended if distal shunts are unsuccesssful and compromised cavernosal artery flow is documented.[66,83] The early implantation of penile prostheses in cases of refractory or recurrent priapism associated with corporal fibrosis and ED have been reported.[66]

The AFUD panel recommendations for management of priapism in patients with SCA include intravenous hydration and parenteral analgesia while preparing for

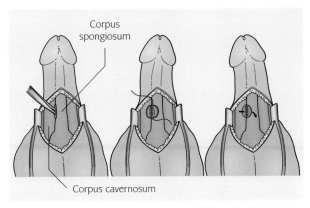

Figure 19. The corporospongiosal shunt. Adapted with permission from Eardley I, Sethia K. *Erectile Dysfunction: Current Investigation and Management*. London: Mosby, 2003.

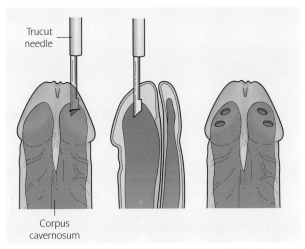

Figure 20. The Winter shunt. Adapted with permission from Eardley I, Sethia K. *Erectile Dysfunction: Current Investigation and Management*. London: Mosby, 2003.

aspiration and irrigation, supplemental oxygen, and exchange transfusion.[66] Initial efforts are directed at relief of pain and anxiety, as well as hydration, with parenteral, hypotonic fluids at 1.5 times maintenance doses. Others report that in the static, hypoxic and acidotic corporal environment, it is unlikely that red cells can reach the area of involvement and question the utility of red cell transfusion.[66,84] Blood volume and viscosity must be closely monitored in SCA patients undergoing exchange transfusion or rapid single unit transfusion, because the risk of cerebrovascular accident, coma and intracranial haemorrhage is significantly increased. If conservative measures are unsuccessful, the management of SCA patients with low-flow priapism is very similar to that for non-SCA patients. "Stuttering" or recurrent, intermittent episodes of painful priapism can be treated with sympathomimetic self-injection and gonadotropin-releasing hormone analogue injection.[85,86]

The treatment for high-flow, arteriogenic priapism consists of conservative alternatives aimed at preservation of sexual function. Mechanical measures may be effective in these patients and consist of external penile compression with perported occlusion of arterial inflow and ice packs. If these approaches are unsuccessful, surgical, pharmacological or radiological treatment may be considered. Surgical and pharmacological interventions have not been very reliable in the treatment of high-flow priapism with maintenance of potency.[86] Selective, transcatheter embolization has been used to occlude arterial inflow with potential preservation of potency in as many as 80% of patients.[87] If embolization is attempted, follow-up duplex Doppler studies are helpful in assessing complete resolution of the arterial fistula and identifying the return of normal cavernosal blood flow.[86]

Peyronie's Disease

Peyronie's disease is a benign condition that causes significant curvature and shortening to the erect penis. This process, produced by scar formation in the fibrous covering or tunica albuginea of the erectile bodies of the penis, occurs most often in men in their late forties and early fifties, and is most common in Caucasians. Men can frequently feel a lump or area of scarring or plaque on top of the shaft of their penis. Symptoms may begin after an injury to the penis during sexual intercourse or from other trauma. Many men notice a period of tenderness in the top portion of the shaft of the penis, most often during erection and worsened by sexual intercourse. Named after François de la Peyronie of France in the mid-18th century, the condition has been reported for many years with a probable increase in prevalence in the past decade. Studies in Olmstead County in Minnesota suggest that 3% of the adult male population over age 40 have scar tissue in their penis from Peyronie's disease.[88] Only about half of these men, however, have significant enough scarring, curvature, ED or penile shortening to require surgical reconstruction. The cause of Peyronie's disease remains a mystery, although many investigators suspect that of the repeated injuries to the penis in men who tend to produce increased amounts of scar tissue, many produce the changes associated with Peyronie's disease. In young men and in men with normal healing properties, when the erect penis is bent, the elastic, fibrous covering of the erectile bodies stretches, recoils and injuries heal without scar tissue. In susceptible men, however, these repeated small traumatic events result in injuries or tears. These injuries produce a small collection of blood or serum between the layers of the tunica albuginea that initiates a cascade of events resulting in the production of collagen of reduced elasticity. These areas heal with the formation of scar tissue, felt as a lump or plaque on top of the shaft of the penis. Some men also have similar changes in the palms of their hands from repeat small trauma, a condition referred to as Dupuytren's contracture. The results of these traumatic events and this scar tissue is a tethering of the penis at the level of the scar, resulting in penile curvature which may vary from minor to severe and incapacitating. Patients may also have indentations in the erect penis called "hourglass" deformity and complain of reduced axial rigidity in that region. They may also suffer from decreased penile length, and erectile difficulties with complete ED or decreased duration of erection. The latter is caused by veno-occlusive incompetence or venous leak ED. Peyronie's disease, while troublesome, is in no way related to sexually transmitted diseases, sexual practices, coital position, or cancer of the penis or other organs. Numerous studies on immunological and genetic associations have proven inconclusive.[89] Risk factors that may increase the possibility of Peyronie's disease include Paget's disease of bone, diabetes, rheumatoid arthritis, use of a vacuum erection device, penile injection, urological instrumentation or catheterization.[90,91] There is a familial association and Peyronie's disease has been reported in identical twins.

Peyronie's disease is often self-limiting, running its course over 12–18 months. During this time, pain usually resolves spontaneously in 4–6 months, curvature may be moderate and plaque size may diminish or soften (see Figure 21). This natural history of Peyronie's disease usually culminates in a stable, non-progressive curvature, which may or may not need further treatment.

Medical therapy

While therapeutic ultrasound was used empirically for this condition 25 years ago, this equipment used often by physical therapy has not demonstrated effectiveness in resolving plaque, curvature, pain and penile narrowing. Similarly, low-dose external beam radiation therapy has

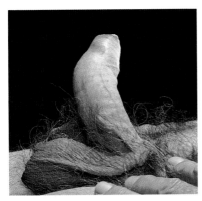

Figure 21. Typical angulation of erection. Reproduced with permission from Eardley I, Sethia K. *Erectile Dysfunction: Current Investigation and Management*. London: Mosby, 2003.

been abandoned as it only treats the penile pain and may result in corporeal fibrosis. Treatment today begins with oral medications in an effort to improve wound healing and soften the scar tissue associated with the plaque. These medications may include vitamin E and Potaba (potassium *para*-aminobenzoate).[91,92] Vitamin E in combination with colchicine, a medication for gout, has also demonstrated effectiveness in some clinical studies.[93] While medications such as tamoxafen and corticosteroids have been used, clear clinical benefit has not been demonstrated. Successful treatment of the plaque with softening, decreased curvature and pain have been demonstrated with direct injection of medications into the Peyronie's plaque. While trials of collagenase have not been successful, verapamil has been widely used with moderate success.[94] The use of alpha-interferon has also been tried with some success. These injection procedures require 6–12 injections directly into the Peyronie's plaque over a 12-week period. Injection therapy, while effective in moderate and mild curvature, is unlikely to be successful in treating severe curvature, calcified plaques or in patients with ED.[93] Trials of topical verapamil gel have also failed, as penetration of the medication into the plaque has been negligible.

During the healing period and the period of evolution of the plaque, it is important for patients to continue to be functional sexually with erectile function and coitus if comfortable. Those men with ED may be effectively treated with an oral PDE5 inhibitor to facilitate erection and improve erectile duration. Many patients can remain sexually active as curvature may be mild to moderate and pain in the penis may resolve quickly. In those patients with continued pain and severe curvature or partner discomfort, surgery may be required to return patient to functional sexual capacity.

Surgical therapy

If medical and expectant therapy fail to resolve the Peyronie's disease and the results of the Peyronie's plaque have produced significantly decreased sexual function, surgery may be an alternative for restoring coital ability. Surgery should be delayed, however, until the disease has stabilized and curvature has not progressed for 6 months or longer.[90] Usually, surgical intervention prior to 18 months after disease onset is not recommended, as progression or resolution may subsequently alter the results of surgical prevention. Surgery is most often used in patients with severe Peyronie's disease that cannot be treated by other, more conservative methods. Significant curvature producing coital discomfort for patient or partner, ED, severe persistent pain and hourglass deformity are all indications for surgical intervention.

Surgical procedures can be divided into three possible alternatives. The first, simplest procedure, termed corporeal plication or the Nesbit procedure (Figure 22), is performed by shortening the penis on the side opposite to the curvature to cancel out the amount of the curve. This procedure, with the least morbidity, is not appropriate for patients with severe curvature or very short penises, as it produces some shortening of the erect penis. Patients continue, however, to have erections and sensation of the penis is usually unaffected by the surgery and ejaculatory ability is preserved. A more direct method for penile straightening is removal or incision (cutting) of the plaque itself,

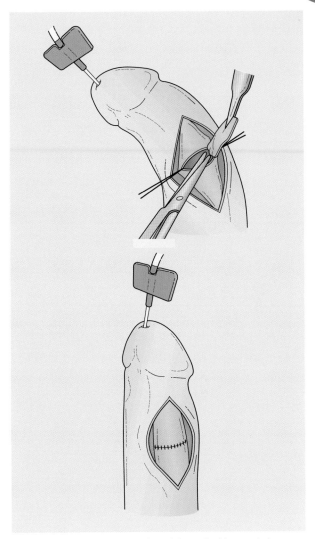

Figure 22. The Nesbit procedure. Adapted with permission from Eardley I, Sethia K. *Erectile Dysfunction: Current Investigation and Management.* London: Mosby, 2003.

straightening of the penis, and replacing the incised or excised tissue of the curved portion of the penis with a

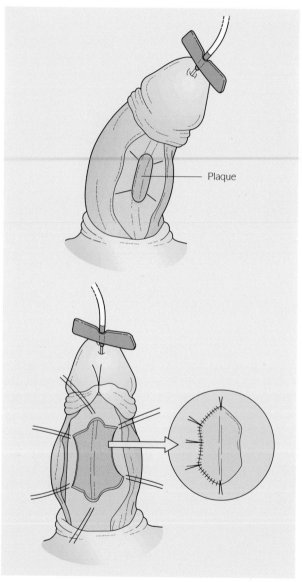

Plaque

Figure 23. The Horton–Devine procedure. Adapted with permission from Eardley I, Sethia K. *Erectile Dysfunction: Current Investigation and Management*. London: Mosby, 2003.

graft.[94,95] This procedure, often termed the Horton–Devine procedure (Figure 23), requires more special surgical ability, experience, and is a longer, more complex surgical procedure. In both of these procedures, an incision similar to a circumcision is usually used with retraction of the skin of the penis to the area of curvature. An erection is created in the operating room using a saline infusion into the corpora cavernosa to allow the surgeon to identify the location and severity of curvature. In the Horton–Devine procedure, the dorsal penile nerves of the top of the penis are dissected away from the curvature and elevated and preserved, an incision is made in the curvature or the plaque itself is removed. The graft inserted may be saphenous vein, undersurface of skin (dermis), tissue from the lining of the testicle (tunica vaginalis), or a packaged material such as cadaveric pericardium or porcine submucosa.[96] All of these graft alternatives provide a flexible, expansile tissue to replace the rigid scarred Peyronie's plaque. While both these procedures are generally successful at straightening the penis and maintaining erectile function, a few patients will notice decreased sensitivity at the tip of their penis, recurrent curvature, continued penile shortening or difficulty with erection.

The third procedure is performed only in those patients with significant ED and deformity caused by Peyronie's disease. In patients with inadequate erection, simple straightening of the penis would not restore the patient's sexual function. As a result, placement of a penile prosthesis can straighten the penis and provide adequate rigidity of the penis for coitus. These devices, which are usually of the inflatable penile prosthesis variety, allow the patient's penis to be straight and rigid enough for intercourse.[96] The urologist implanting this prosthesis may perform a penile modelling procedure once the prosthesis is placed, to complete the penile straightening. This latter procedure, which breaks up the scar tissue fibres of the Peyronie's plaque during surgery, will enhance the straightening of the penis and improve ultimate postoperative result. Risks of this procedure, in addition to those mentioned previously, include infection of the prosthesis, mechanical malfunction or prosthesis leak, and repeat curvature. In a recent study, patients with Peyronie's disease and penile prostheses had high overall satisfaction rates and more than 80% of patients stated that they would undergo penile prosthesis again for treatment of their Peyronie's disease.[97] A similar study investigating patients undergoing plaque incision and grafting without prosthesis demonstrated a more than 90% patient satisfaction rate.[95]

Summary

Peyronie's disease is an uncommon condition whose prevalence is rising. The symptoms include penile curvature, shortening, pain and ED. Peyronie's disease should be treated initially conservatively with watchful waiting or medication with a high expectation for improvement or resolution. In those patients with continued erectile difficulties from curvature or inadequate erections, surgical procedures designed to care for Peyronie's disease have been refined and are usually successful, with high patient satisfaction outcomes.

Diabetes, Hypertension, Coronary Artery Disease and Erectile Dysfunction

Diabetes mellitus and erectile dysfunction

Diabetes is an important cause of ED, and ED is common in men with diabetes . It may occur in 35% of all men with diabetes, increasing to >50% over the age of 50 years and further still with increasing age.[98]

ED can cause significant loss of self-esteem and reduction in quality of life, which may reduce the motivation of men to control the diabetes itself.

Active screening or at least a good awareness programme should be practiced by healthcare professionals involved in diabetes care.

Diabetes is a chronic metabolic disorder with many complications and associated factors that predispose to ED. There are therefore many reasons why men with diabetes have a high incidence of ED and these are outlined in Table 30.

Type 1 (insulin-dependent) diabetes

In type 1 diabetes, ED is associated with the following factors:
- Age of patient.
- Duration of diabetes.
- Degree of control (level of glycosylated haemoglobin).
- Presence of microvascular disease.
- Cardiovascular risk factors and/or disease.

Type 2 (non-insulin-dependent) diabetes

In type 2 diabetes, the above factors also apply but cardiovascular risk factors and disease probably predominate.

Table 30. Factors leading to the high incidence of ED in diabetes
Stress of living with a chronic disease
Metabolic effects of hyperglycaemia and excessive protein glycosylation
Penile disorders: balanitis, phimosis, Peyronie's disease
Premature ageing and degeneration of corpora cavernosal smooth muscle
Endothelial dysfunction
Microvascular complications and smooth muscle myopathy
Sensory and autonomic neuropathy
Macrovascular disease and its risk factors, treatments and consequences
Hypertension and its treatment

Targets of diabetes control

Modern targets of diabetes control are now very strict and aimed at reducing both microvascular disease and cardiovascular risk (Table 31).

The achievement of such targets often requires multiple drug therapy, some of which itself may be associated with an increased incidence of ED. Such drug regimes include:
- Oral hypoglycaemic agents.
- Multiple drug antihypertensive regimes.
- Lipid-lowering agents.

When choosing antihypertensive drugs, it is advisable to ask men about erectile function and be sensitive to their needs in this respect.

Angiotensin-converting enzyme (ACE) inhibitors, angiotensin-2 antagonists, and sympathetic alpha-adrenoreceptor blockers and vasodilators are probably the least likely to have a major effect on ED. Beta-blockers and diuretics, on the other hand, are most likely to have an adverse effect.

ED occurs much earlier in the course of type 2 diabetes. Indeed, ED may be the presenting symptom. All patients presenting with ED should be screened for undiagnosed

Table 31. Targets in diabetes mellitus management	
Blood pressure	<140/80
Glycaemic control	Glycosylated haemoglobin (HBA1c) <7%
Lipids	Cholesterol/HDL ratio <5 LDL <3 Triglycerides <2.2

diabetes. Up to 16% of men presenting with ED may have undiagnosed diabetes.

Aetiology and treatments
Aetiology
ED in diabetic men may occur due to the presence of any of the causes of ED in the non-diabetic man. It is probably multifactorial in most diabetic men.

Recent interest has focused on the structure and function of the smooth muscle and endothelium of the corpora cavernosa themselves. Degeneration and endothelial cell dysfunction related to advanced glycation products adversely affecting the activated NO pathways may be of particular significance.[99,100]

There is an increased incidence of Peyronie's disease in diabetes (often in association with Dupuytren's contractures in the hands, further demonstrating collagen degeneration).

Because of the above factors, the ED suffered by the diabetic man is often severe and complete.

Treatments for ED and the diabetic man
All treatments are suitable for the man with diabetes and ED, and the choice should be based on availability, suitability and personal preference, as with the non-diabetic man.

Because of the severity of the ED, treatments may not be quite as effective, but most men can be helped by one or other of the available therapies.

Hypertension and erectile dysfunction

Hypertension is a common condition estimated to affect up to 41% of men and 33% of women if >140/90 is used as the definition. ED is more common and more severe in men with hypertension and ED of a moderate or severe degree may affect up to 60%.[101] Although antihypertensive drugs are often cited as the cause, hypertension itself is a significant aetiological factor.

Factors related to the high incidence of ED in hypertensive men include:

- Arteriosclerosis.
- Endothelial cell dysfunction.
- Impaired NO–cGMP pathway.
- Excessive sympathetic nervous system activity and tone.
- High incidence of other cardiovascular risk factors – diabetes, smoking, dyslipidaemia.
- Antihypertensive drugs.
- Excess alcohol.

Antihypertensive drugs may exacerbate or cause ED in men who are already susceptible. This may occur as a result of the following actions of these drugs:

- Central effects on the brain.
- Reduced peripheral penile perfusion.
- Adverse effects on endothelial cell function and NO–cGMP pathways.

Treatment for hypertension should be tailored as much as possible to suit the individual man. Men should be questioned about erectile function and practitioners should be sensitive to this issue when initiating or increasing treatment.

The drugs with the lowest incidence of ED as an unwanted effect are perhaps:

- Alpha-adrenergic blocking vasodilators.
- ACE inhibitors.
- Angiotensin-2 antagonists.

Altering antihypertensive drugs in men with ED

Modifying antihypertensive drug regimes in men with ED unfortunately does not often meet with success unless there is a definite temporal association between the onset of ED and the taking of a particular drug.

All men presenting with ED should be screened for hypertension.

Coronary artery disease and erectile dysfunction

There remains a centuries old persistent myth that sex is dangerous and may lead to sudden "death on the job". This concern continues to worry patients, their partners and some healthcare professionals, despite a wealth of reassuring evidence to the contrary.

Many men with coronary artery disease (CAD) will suffer with ED and many men with ED will suffer from CAD, although this may occult.

Issues that need to be considered in the context of ED and CAD include:

- Importance of ED in men with CAD.
- Importance of CAD in men with ED.
- Cardiovascular disease and risks of sexual activity.
- Myocardial infarction, sex and rehabilitation.
- Safety of treatments for ED in men with CAD.

Erectile dysfunction is common in men with known cardiovascular disease (Table 32).

Previously undiagnosed cardiovascular disease is common in men with ED and includes:

- Diabetes.
- Hypertension.
- Ischaemic heart disease.
- Peripheral vascular disease.

Table 32. Incidence of ED in men with cardiovascular disease	
Untreated hypertension	17%
Treated hypertension	25–60%
Diabetes mellitus	>50%
Post-myocardial infarction	40%

Studies suggest that the incidence of ED increases with the severity of CAD (Table 33).[102] The causes of ED in CAD are likely to be multifactorial and are outlined in Table 34.

The risks of sex: is it dangerous?

Sexual activity under normal circumstances involves physical and emotional exercise, but is not unduly strenuous compared with other everyday activities. This has been well summarized by Hellerstein:[103]

"Sex is brief, low frequency and modest in its physical demands…"

"Comparable cardiovascular stresses are encountered frequently during the daily performance of the customary low energy requiring occupations of the typical hypokinetic, unfit middle aged man."

Table 33. Occult coronary artery disease in men with ED
80% multiple vascular risk factors
Exercise ECG abnormal in 28
Severe coronary artery disease on angiography – 6
Moderate – 2
Single vessel – 7

Table 34. Causes of ED in men with coronary artery disease
Fear, anxiety, depression
Shared risk factors: lipids, smoking, diabetes, hypertension
Atherosclerosis
Drug treatments
Partner factors

Risks

Although the risk of myocardial infarction is increased in the 2-hour period following sexual activity, this risk is very low. The risks are shown in Table 35. Overall, the risk of sexual activity causing a myocardial infarction is <1% of cases. This statistic should be reassuring.[104]

Relative risks are also low (see Table 36), and the benefits of regular physical activity and fitness clearly apparent.

Physiological cost of sexual activity

The physiological cost of sexual activity is similar to many ordinary daily activities. It can be measured by the effect on heart rate and blood pressure or as the metabolic equivalent of the task (MET). MET is measured as the relative energy demand of oxygen usage at rest, which is

Table 35. Sex and myocardial infarction: absolute risks	
No previous CVS event	1/1,000,000/hour daily activity
	2/1,000,000/hour post coitus
Previous CVS event	10/1,000,000/hour daily activity
	30/1,000,000/hour post coitus

Table 36. Sex and myocardial infarction: relative risks	
All men	2.5
Prior myocardial infarction	2.9
Sedentary	3.0
Physically active and "fit"	1.2

approximately 3.5 ml of oxygen/kg body weight/minute. These effects are shown in Tables 37 and 38.[105]

Sexual dysfunction following myocardial infarction (MI)
Men and their partners may be concerned about resuming sexual activity after a myocardial infarction. They may be reluctant and embarrassed to seek advice. Advice regarding

Table 37. Effects of sexual activity on heart rate and blood pressure	
Time	5–15 minutes
Heart rate	120–150
On beta-blocker	80
Systolic blood pressure	150–180
Peak stress	3–5 minutes
Equivalent to 3–4 minutes Bruce protocol exercise ECG stress test	

Table 38. Comparative physiological effects of sex versus other activities (metabolic equivalents of the tasks, METs)	
Activity	MET score
Sex	2–6
Walking on level 20 minutes	3–4
Golf	4–5
Gardening	3–5
Light housework	2–4
3–4 minutes Bruce ETT	4–6

sexual activity should be a routine part of rehabilitation following myocardial infarction or any other significant cardiovascular event.

Causes of ED after an MI include:

- Fear, anxiety, depression.
- Cardiac symptoms.
- Partner concern.
- Drugs treatments.
- Pre-existing ED.

Management

In considering ED post-MI, the objectives should be to restore the couple to their preinfarct level of sexual activity. Failure to do so usually correlates better with fear and anxiety than with the severity of the infarct itself.

Management should include:

- Sensitive discussion and advice.
- Consideration of the circumstances and partner.
- Reassurance of the patient and partner.

It may be useful to discuss the Masters and Johnson sensate focusing exercises, which may help reassure couples and improve communication. Masturbation may reassure men and their partners that orgasm can be survived!

Risk assessment

It is important to compare the energies of likely sexual activity with other, tolerated everyday activities and to grade cardiovascular risk. Risk can be graded according to cardiovascular status. Such a grading has been agreed in published consensus statements and is shown in Table 39.[106]

Treatments in the patient with cardiovascular disease

Assuming grading and appropriate treatment of the cardiovascular disease has been completed, then ED

Table 39. Management recommendations according to cardiovascular risk

Categories of CVD	Management recommendations
Management recommendations – low risk	
Asymptomatic, <3 major risk factors for CAD – excluding age and gender	Primary care management
Controlled hypertension	Consider all first-line therapies
Minimal/mild, stable angina	Reassess at regular intervals (6–12 months)
Post-successful coronary revascularization	
Uncomplicated MI (<6–8 weeks ago)	
Mild valvular disease	
CHF (grade1)	
Management recommendations – intermediate risk	
Asymptomatic but >3 major risk factors	Consider specialist CVA testing (e.g. ETT, Echo)
For CAD, excluding gender	Restratification into high or low risk based on further assessment
Moderate, stable angina	
Recent MI (within last 2–6 weeks)	
LVD/CHF (grade 1, 2)	
Non-cardiac sequelae of atherosclerotic disease (e.g. CVA, peripheral vascular disease)	
Management recommendations – high risk	
Severe or unstable or refractory angina	Priority referral for specialized CVA management
Uncontrolled hypertension (SBP >180 mmHg)	Treatment for sexual dysfunction to be deferred until cardiac condition stabilized and dependent on specialist recommendations
Recent MI or CVA (within last 14 days)	
LVD, CHF (grade 3, 4)	
High risk arrhythmias	
Hypertrophic cardiomyopathy	
Moderate/severe valvular disease	

CAD, coronary artery disease; CHF, congestive heart failure; CVA, stroke; LVD, left ventricular dysfunction; MI, myocardial infarction; SABP, systolic blood pressure.

treatment can be actioned. All treatment modalities should be considered. Treatment concerns include potential problems with:

- Warfarin.
- Nitrates

Warfarin is a relative contraindication if considering a vacuum device (petechiae, haematoma) or MUSE (bleeding).

Nitrate drugs are a contraindication if considering PDE5 inhibitor oral treatment. Nitrates are not only used for angina, but also for other medical indications and for recreational use, and this should be remembered. A list of available nitrate drugs and other nitric acid donors is included in Appendix 1.

PDE5 inhibitors and nitrates

The effects of using Viagra are shown in Table 40. If using nitrates, the following applies:

- Absolute contraindication.
- Discuss alternative ED treatments.
- Consider discontinuing nitrates.

Nitrates are not of prognostic significance in patients with CAD, but are a symptomatic treatment. In many instances they can be discontinued or an alternative anti-anginal agent such as a calcium channel blocker or beta-blocker substituted.

Table 40. Viagra (and other PDE5 inhibitors) and coronary artery disease
Well tolerated
Effective in 60–80% of men
Similar cardiovascular effect to nitrates
No effect on heart rate
No effect on resting or exercise ECG
Modest fall in blood pressure: systolic 8–10 mmHg, diastolic 4–6 mmHg
No increased incidence of death, MI or stroke

Short-acting nitrates should not be used within 12 hours of a PDE5 inhibitor or vice versa. Long-acting nitrates should not be used within 1 week of a PDE5 inhibitor or vice versa.

A reasonable course of action to take in this situation is shown in Table 41.

Table 41. Coronary artery disease, nitrates, Viagra and ED
Angina troublesome:
Consider calcium antagonist and/or beta-blocker
Investigate with exercise test and echocardiogram. Refer to cardiology
Defer ED treatment
No angina:
Stop long-acting nitrate for 1 week
Encourage exercise
Advise regarding short-acting nitrates
If no angina -- prescribe Viagra. Ban use of short-acting nitrate
Angina recurs:
Prescribe calcium channel blocker and/or beta-blocker
Refer to cardiology if no response
Start Viagra when/if angina free

Ejaculatory Disorders

Disorders of ejaculation are amongst the most common sexual complaints yet are the most difficult to adequately treat. Of the physiological processes of sexual function, ejaculation is one of the least well understood.

Physiology of ejaculation

Ejaculation can be divided into two processes, emission and ejaculation. This event, when tied to the emotional and psychological event, is termed orgasm in the male. Emission occurs when fluid is deposited in the posterior urethra. This ejaculate fluid originates from the epididymis, vas deferens, seminal vesicles and prostate. Indeed, the seminal vesicles contribute the majority of the ejaculate volume and sperm are added from the ampullae of the vas deferens close to the prostate. The sequence of ejaculatory events includes pre-ejaculation, where the vesical neck closes, followed by deposition of fluid from the seminal tract into the posterior urethra. The fluid is forcefully mixed after secretion and subsequently is forcibly expelled from the urethra by rhythmic contractions of the perineal muscles, including the ischiocavernosus and bulbocavernosus muscles.[104] If climax is accompanied by an absence of fluid at the penile meatus, it is termed aspermia. Azoospermia in distinction is the absence of sperm in the ejaculate.

Normally, ejaculate volume is 1.5–5 ml, with 80% from the seminal vesicles, 10% from the prostate, and 10% from the ampullae of the vas deferens and small amounts of fluid from the periurethral glands, including Cowper's glands.[107] The first 0.5 ml of ejaculate contains the highest concentration of sperm, as well as zinc, citrate and prostatic acid phosphatase. The seminal vesicles provide the final portion of the volume and contain the highest amounts of fructose. An ejaculate without fructose suggests obstruction of the seminal vesicles or ejaculatory ducts.

Ejaculation is under the neural control of the sympathetic and somatic nerves, with emission a sympathetic function and ejaculation a somatic function. The efferent sympathetic nerves arise from the T10–L2 segments of the thoracolumbar spine.[107] These segments give rise to the superior hypogastric plexus, which innervates the prostate, bladder base, vasa and seminal vesicles. The somatic supply of ejaculation and expulsion of fluid is from the S2–S4 level via the perineal branch of the pudendal nerve.

Classification and clinical evaluation

Ejaculatory dysfunction may be classified as primary (lifelong) or secondary (acquired). The latter is far more common in clinical practice. Premature ejaculation is defined as ejaculation in less than 1 minute or before partner satisfaction in at least 50% of attempts.[108,109] Premature ejaculation is more common in younger men and was the most prevalent sexual dysfunction reported in the National Health and Social Life Survey (NHSLS) by Laumann et al.,[110] accounting for more than 35% of sexual dysfunction. The aetiology of premature ejaculation remains controversial and clearly has a psychological or learned component in most men.[111] Evaluation of men with retrograde ejaculation should include a thorough history to identify risk factors such as diabetes, urological surgery, nerve injury or hypogonadism. Physical examination should focus on neurological examination, secondary male sex characteristics and urological examination of penis, testes and prostate. Laboratory studies that may be helpful are blood glucose and hormone profile, including total and free testosterone.

Treatment of premature ejaculation

Treatment of premature ejaculation is primarily medical.[112,113] Psychological treatment was the mainstay of treatment in years past, when methods of psychological training and conditioning were popular. Use of progressive relaxation techniques and passive or less aggressive coital techniques are used by many psychologists with little long-term success. Psychological counselling is quite helpful as an adjunct to medical or topical therapy, and the combination of these modalities may lead to more rapid and lingering duration of success. The "squeeze" or "pinch" technique, whereby the erect penis is squeezed firmly below the glans penis (at the corona penis), can be used and is carried out for 15–30 seconds to create a temporary neuropathy and desensitize the glans penis.[114] This procedure was widely used, but infrequently effective. Medical treatment can be topical or systemic. The former includes use of a condom or local anaesthetic to decrease glans sensitivity.[115] Lidocaine gel (2%) or EMLA cream (2.5% lidocaine/2.5% prilocaine) have been applied 15–30 minutes prior to coitus and have been shown to increase the time to ejaculation in more than 75% of men treated.[115] Patients must use a condom or wash the penile surface thoroughly before coitus to avoid vaginal absorption of the anaesthetic medication. The most effective treatment is the recently reported use of selective serotonin reuptake inhibitors (SSRIs). These medications may be associated with retarded or absent ejaculation in patients treated for depression. Placebo-controlled trials have documented the effectiveness of these agents.[112,113] While the choice of SSRI varies, they are administered in a daily dose until ejaculation returns to normal, then as needed before coitus. While sertraline was the first agent used, experience with other SSRIs has produced excellent results. Table 42 lists the

Table 42. Medications for premature ejaculation		
Drug	**Dosage (mg)**	**Frequency**
Paroxetine	20	Daily
Fluoxetine	20	Daily
Sertraline	50	Daily
Clomipramine	25	Daily

agents, dosage and frequency of administration. Adverse events from SSRIs include anxiety, gastrointestinal distress, drowsiness and anticholinergic effects.

The tricyclic antidepressant agent clomipramine has also been used in trials with some success.[112] Daily use of 25 mg may be used in patients refractory to SSRI treatment. This agent has significant side-effects, such as anticholinergic effects, gastrointestinal disturbance and drowsiness. Sildenafil has been used for premature ejaculation with some success.[116] PDE5 agents may assist in erectile duration and provide some patient confidence in the ability to maintain an erection long enough for satisfactory coitus with his partner.

Treatment of retrograde ejaculation

Retrograde ejaculation is aspermia or decreased ejaculate volume caused by deficient closure of the bladder neck. Causes include the peripheral neuropathy of diabetes mellitus and other conditions, medications such as alpha-blockers used to treat LUTS and transurethral surgery such as TURP. Spinal cord injury with lesions at or below the T10–L2 region may also lead to retrograde ejaculation. The incidence of retrograde ejaculation is not well studied, but 0.7% of men with male factor infertility, more than 30% of diabetics and 25–30% of men following TURP will suffer premature ejaculation. Men undergoing retroperitoneal lymphadenectomy and lumbar disc fusion are also at high risk.[116]

Treatment is likewise difficult. Surgical treatment has been described, but is rarely successful. Medications, which may improve or resolve retrograde ejaculation, are unreliable. Alpha-adrenergic agonist agents are the first agents to use, although adverse events may outweigh therapeutic effect. Medication may be given before coitus or on a regular daily schedule.[117] Table 43 lists some of the agents often employed for retrograde ejaculation.

In men with male factor infertility who are unable to conceive because of retrograde ejaculation, harvesting of

Table 43. Medications for the treatment of retrograde ejaculation	
Agents given 1–2 hours before coitus	
Pseudoephedrine	120 mg
Phenylephrine	
Ephedrine	30–60 mg
Agents given daily	
Pseudoephedrine	60 mg qid
Phenylpropanolamine	75 mg bid
Chlorpheniramine	bid
Brompheniramine	bid
Imipramine	25 mg bid

sperm from the bladder following ejaculation with sperm washing and artificial insemination of the female partner is often successful. In spinal cord-injured men who cannot ejaculate, electrical stimulation through a rectal probe can be useful in selected patients.[118]

Retarded or anejaculation

Primary anejaculation is a rare condition occurring in less than 1% of men. Treatment is primarily through psychotherapy and is often unsuccessful.[107] Stimulation of ejaculation with vibratory stimuli or electro-ejaculation may be used for obtaining sperm for insemination and ultimately trans-scrotal sperm harvesting may be necessary in some patients.

Retarded ejaculation and anejaculation are especially troublesome symptoms most common in older men. As men age, ejaculatory frequency, volume and force decline naturally. Similarly, the glans penis sensation is reduced in older men. They often require more stimulation for a longer duration for successful ejaculation. Adding neuropathic changes, hypogonadism or SSRI medications will further retard ejaculation.[107] SSRI-associated retarded ejaculation may be improved through change in antidepressant medication if possible.[119] Non-SSRI agents such as serzone and trazodone may allow return of ejaculation with continued depression treatment. These agents are not as successful in treating men with depression as the SSRI medications and a change in the class of antidepressant may not be possible in men with moderate to severe depression.[119] Similarly, use of PDE5 inhibitors such as sildenafil will often allow an erection of adequate duration for older men to successfully ejaculate. No specific drug therapy is currently available for treatment of these patients.

Haematospermia

Haematospermia is an infrequent association of ejaculation and may be caused by prostatitis, seminal vesiculitis, prostatic calculi or rarely prostate cancer. Haematospermia is usually a painless condition of brown or dark semen in men over age 50. If painful, the usual cause is prostatitis, but may be ejaculatory duct obstruction or prostatic calculi.[120] Evaluation should include a digital rectal examination, urine culture, prostatic secretion culture after voiding and prostate-specific antigen. If prostate cancer or ejaculatory duct obstruction is suspected, transrectal ultrasound may be useful.[121]

Future Developments

The last decade has witnessed the physiology and molecular biology of erectile function and ED elucidated and translational research from these studies have led to the understanding of the physiology of erection and also significant progress in the diagnosis and treatment of men with erectile dysfunction (ED). Basic science laboratory investigation has clarified the anatomy, physiology, and pharmacology of the corpus cavernosum as well as the neurophysiology and vascular physiology of erectile function.

Investigation of the subcellular function of corpus cavernosum smooth muscle and its nerve supply have led to a clear understanding of the neurotransmitters and their effects on corpus cavernosum smooth muscle tissue. A number of these molecules are involved in smooth muscle contraction as well as relaxation. A balance of contraction and relaxation mechanisms is necessary for maintenance of penile flaccidity as well as erection. Contractile elements include such molecules as endothelin-1, prostaglandin F2, and epinephrine. Counteracting these contractile agents may also facilitate erectile function. The use of such agents as oral phentolamine may improve erectile function by overcoming smooth muscle contractile elements.

Pharmacological treatment of ED

The next decades are likely to see significant additions to the armamentarium of physicians and the treatment of ED. Newer PDE5 agents are already poised for launch in the US and are available in the European and other international markets. Novel CNS agents are available in Europe and newer more selective CNS agents are being developed. Similarly advances in androgen treatment are being evaluated along with newer methods of hormonal evaluation. In the more invasive choices newer injectable, topical, and surgical alternatives have been introduced and are being refined.

Androgen treatment

Deficient testosterone and androgen function in laboratory animals results in decreased corpus cavernosum smooth muscle contraction. Delivery systems in patients with hypogonadism or androgen deficiency in the ageing male (ADAM), however, have been suboptimal. Currently the efficient diagnosis of ADAM is difficult and frequently late in the course of the condition. Identification of the ADAM syndrome is principally on the basis of symptoms followed by laboratory studies identifying low levels of testosterone and other androgens. Questionnaires are being developed and are in their early stages to help identify men with ADAM. While early in their development and of high sensitivity but poor specificity, these questionnaires may be successfully used when subsequent iterations of these instruments are available. Oral androgen replacement therapy available in the US has resulted in rapid hepatitic metabolism, hepatotoxicity but no specific improvement or increase in serum testosterone. Other oral agents available in Canada and Europe are more successful with less toxicity. These agents including testosterone undecenoate enhance serum testosterone without the toxicity of methyl testosterone alternatives.[8] The field of testosterone replacement, however, has been revolutionized by the introduction of topical application devices and techniques. Transdermal patches to provide testosterone supplementation using polymeric membrane patches permit the sustained release of testosterone for at least 22 hours. These transdermal patches that began as scrotal applications are now available for applications elsewhere on the body over areas of adequate muscle mass. Reproducing the normal diurnal curve, the maximum testosterone levels with these patches occurs early in the morning and declines late in the evening similar to the physiologic production of testosterone under the control of pituitary hormones. While these patches are clearly more expensive than oral or injectable testosterone supplementation alternatives, their physiologic pattern of administration may provide advantages over oral or injectable testosterone treatment.[10]

More recent developments in the treatment of ADAM have been necessitated by dermatitis caused by some of the patch systems. The development of testosterone gels (Andro Gel and Testim) has improved the transdermal route of administration by improving ease of use and decreasing the skin eruptions while maintaining effectiveness. Different from testosterone patches, however, testosterone gel is applied each morning after shower with expected peak levels at 8 to 10 a.m. declining until the next application the following morning. Similar to the patches, however, this pattern replicates the normal diurnal physiologic testosterone production curve. Caveats to these gels include maintaining a dry surface for 2 hours following application to allow absorption, avoiding contact of the applied gel to a female partner for at least 2 hours. Follow-up should include monitoring serum testosterone levels 4 weeks following initial treatment and every 6 months afterwards. Annual evaluation of PSA, lipid profile, liver enzymes, and blood count are also suggested to avoid some of the potential side-effects of testosterone replacement therapy. The effectiveness of testosterone gel appears to be equivalent to that of testosterone patches. Andro Gel is available in 1% solution, in 2.5, and 5 g packets while Testim is available as a 1% gel, in 5 g and 10 g tubes. Patients may need more than one packet or tube each day to maintain normal testosterone levels and levels should be followed carefully by serum blood levels. Newer gel agents are being investigated including a dihydrotestosterone (DHT) preparation that may provide direct application of the activated form of testosterone and may be useful in both male and female sexual dysfunction.

Significant research continues on the effects of other testicular and non-testicular androgens including Androstenedione and Dehydroepiandrosterone (DHEA) early studies show that these agents affect androgen receptors in the prostate and the corpora cavernosa. An Austrian study suggests that DHEA deficiency can be associated with decreased libido and sexual function in some men. Whether replacement of these adrenal and non-testicular androgen molecules will improve sexual function and ED is uncertain. A better understanding of the hormonal influences on sexual function is one of the frontiers of investigation in the 21st century.

Oral agents

Oral agents were unreliable prior to the development of the currently available PDE5 agents. Newer oral agents are now available for clinical use and newer agents are in various stages of clinical trials and early development. The 21st century will see many new pharmacologic approaches to the treatment of ED. Sildenafil, the first approved oral agent for clinical use introduced in 1998 has revolutionized the evaluation and treatment of ED.[30,122] Several novel PDE5 inhibitors are now available including vardenafil and tadalafil. Tanake Seiyaku is developing a new short acting PDE5 (TA1790) and several nasal, sublingual, and topical PDE5s are being tried.

Centrally acting agents

Apomorphine (Uprima) stimulates postsynaptic dopamine receptors in the hypothalamus and is effective as a precoital oral agent. Currently available only in Europe, apomorphine is under review by the US Food and Drug Administration. Apomorphine has long been known to be erectogenic and is now thought to stimulate the D1 and D2 dopamine receptors in the midbrain. While it is likely that the D2 receptors are inhibitory, the D1 receptors appear to be associated with erection. Previously, apomorphine was used in the laboratory to stimulate erection but had significant side-effects including nausea and vomiting. Heaton *et al.* however were able to formulate a sublingual administration that has preserved the erectogenic activity while decreasing noxious side-effects. Nastech and Brittania Pharmaceuticals are using a nasal route of administration to enhance speed of onset without increasing adverse events.

Newer CNS agents have been used in early clinical trials with good efficacy and fewer side-effects. Melanotan 2 (MSHII) being developed by Palatin Technologies, as PT141 is a non-selective melanocortin receptor agonist. PT141 currently undergoing phase three pharmacologic trials appears to produce erectile function mediated through receptors in the brain. This agent that mimics the activity of ACTH and Alpha MSH may improve erectile function in both cycogenic and organic erectile dysfunction. Its activity, similar to apomorphine, appears to have fewer adverse side-effects while preserving central nervous system erectile function. Taken 30 minutes before coitus, PT141 has been effective in as many as 80% of sildenafil failures in Phase II trials.

An additional central nervous system agent is an isomer of sibutramine, a popular weight loss agent that has been developed for oral use with reasonable early results. Side-effects are few and similar agents may lead to CNS agents with good efficacy and tolerability. These agents would be well suited for patients taking nitrates and might assist men and women with arousal disorders, a significant challenge in the treatment of both male and female sexual problems.

NO donors may be useful alone or as combination products in enhancing erections. l-arginine and yohimbine have been investigated in Italy with erectogenic effect and oral phentolamine, a non-specific alpha blocker called Bimexes is being used in Mexico for the treatment of ED.

Injectable agents

The use of injectable vasoactive agents for the stimulation of erectile function began in 1983 with the dramatic presentation by Brindley at the American Urologic Association Meeting in Los Vegas, Nevada.[14] Following his stimulating discussion and graphic demonstration of the effectiveness of intracavernosal injected pharmacoactive agents, the international urological community began the widespread use of these agents in patients of all ages. Combinations of injectable agents are widely used internationally. A combination of phentolamine and VIP has been approved in several European countries. This combination product, called Invicorp® (Senetec), has responses equivalent to PGE_1 without penile pain and aching. Moxisylyte, a selective alpha-1 receptor blocking substance, has also been approved for use in several European countries.[29] This agent, which relaxes smooth muscle in a fashion similar to phentolamine, has a reported success rate of 70% at doses of 10–30 mg. Adverse events include prolonged erection (1%) and corpus cavernosum fibrosis (1.5%). Comparisons between Moxisylyte and PGE_1 demonstrate stronger penile rigidity and higher success for PGE_1, but decreased penile pain and discomfort with moxisylyte.[29]

Combination therapy

As newer pharmacological agents are introduced and their efficacy and safety confirmed as single agents, the natural progression for patients that fail or cannot tolerate single agents is to try a course of combination therapy. Small series with combinations of sildenafil and MUSE have been reported with excellent success and no significant additional adverse events. Significantly, in these selected patients, no prolonged erections or priapism were reported. Other combinations with penile implants and MUSE have also demonstrated good results in men with "cold glans" decreased arousal and penile prosthesis malfunction. In both combination schemes, low doses of MUSE appear to be effective. Anecdotally, sildenafil has been used successfully for increasing penile engorgement in men with penile implants.

Future directions include a continuation of these combinations with a topical or local acting agent with a CNS agent. This type of combination therapy may permit each agent to be given at a lower dose than single therapy and decrease the adverse events of each agent.

Gene therapy

Gene therapy for the treatment of ED may be one of the ideal locations for the use of this novel and ground-breaking technology. Already, many investigators have used NOS or potassium channel opening agents transfected by gene therapy to treat *in vivo* ED with good success. These experiments have been used in diabetes, vasculogenic and trauma models of ED with high success rates. These treatments *in vivo*, however, require redosing every 1–3 months by direct injection. In the future, therefore, a diabetic man with ED might have to see his physician three to four times yearly for an injection that would result in a restoration of his normal ability to obtain and maintain an erection. Other types of gene therapy may also be useful in restoring androgen production, sensitivity and reducing ADAM.

Penile prosthesis

Recent developments in penile prosthesis design have included efforts to decrease the incidence of infection-associated failures. Both American Medical Systems (AMS) and Mentor Corporation have introduced concepts that will decrease these tragic complications. While the Mentor device coating Resist™ has yet to be introduced to the market, this hydrophilic coating is similar to that used on stents and catheters. The Resist™ coating has been used *in vitro* and in clinical trials with commonly used topical

Table 44. ED treatment types		
	Facilitators	**Stimulators**
Central	Testosterone DHEA	Apomorphine Dopamine agonists and reuptake inhibitors
Peripheral	PDE5 inhibitors Phentolamine (Vasomax) Testosterone	Alprostadil Papaverine Phentolamine Forskolin
Devices	Penile implants, vacuum devices	

antibiotic solutions to decrease the early adherence of bacteria to the implanted device. This coating results in a longer-lasting adherence of antibiotic agents and has been reported to last 24–36 hours and result in fewer *Staphyloccus*-related colonizations and infections. As a result of the hydrophilic properties, bacteria are less likely to adhere to the surface early in the postoperative period. Its true effectiveness awaits formal clinical trials and clinical experience. The AMS three-piece inflatable prostheses are now available with a coating called InhibiZone®. This coating consists of a combination of minocycline and rifampin, which remains on the implant fabric for up to 3 days. This combination antibiotic coating is targeted at the most common infection related pathogens, the Gram-positive staphylococci, such as *S. epidermidis*. Early postoperative results have demonstrated an advantage in both first and repeat implants compared with historical and contemporary implant infection rates for prostheses implanted without InhibiZone®.

The AMS prostheses have also been redesigned to include a coating of paralene to increase the tensile strength of the silicone elastomer from which they are made. This redesign is aimed at further reducing the mechanical malfunction rate and the life of the devices. These devices currently have an expected 5-year survival in excess of 90%.

Summary

With newer novel methods for the treatment of ED, urologists and other healthcare providers can offer men with ED a variety of solutions suited to their pathophysiology, aetiology and personal needs. Because many patients fail to maintain treatment with injectable and more invasive therapeutic alternatives, oral treatment and combinations of agents appear to be the best method for treatment of men who do not respond to simple oral therapy.123 Heaton et al.124 have suggested a method for consideration of pharmacological treatment of ED including central and peripheral medications which produce stimulation or facilitation of erectile function (Table 44). By applying this grid to a decision tree once multiple oral and injectable medications are available, urologists with a knowledge and expertise in ED may design therapeutic programmes for individual patients refractory to simple single oral therapy.

Frequently Asked Questions and Misconceptions

Is there an age limit beyond which ED treatments are contraindicated or unwarranted?

ED occurs increasingly with age and is therefore very common in the very elderly. Partners are also likely to be of a similar age. Sexual activity and the requirement of sexual satisfaction usually falls with age, but there are a significant number of men for whom it remains of importance. There are no particular age-related contraindications to treatments, but an individualized and sensitive approach is required to assess suitability. This will involve assessment of associated conditions and particularly mental and physical aptitude to ensure safety. Treatments can be very successful and, as with younger people, can lead to significant improvements in quality of life.

Which patients should be referred for surgical treatment, i.e. consideration for a penile prosthesis?

The following might be considered factors warranting referral:

- Congenital or acquired anatomical abnormalities.
- Severe corpora cavernosal fibrosis – post-injection therapy, Peyronie's, etc.
- Failure of other treatments.
- Patient preference and unwillingness to try, or persevere with, other treatments.

Which patients should be referred for psychosexual therapy?

Most men with ED will have have some relevant psychological factors that either precipitate or potentiate their problem. If the underlying cause is predominantly a physical one, it is reasonable for the general practitioner or physician to recommend a physical treatment while also discussing the psychological aspects in general terms. General counselling is as important an adjunct to physical treatments in "physical ED" as physical treatments are to psychological treatments in "psychological ED". Physical treatment, although effective in restoring an erect penis, does not treat the underlying cause in men with psychological causes and the following people should be referred for specialist psychosexual treatment:

- Men in whom the cause is predominantly psychological and not helped by general counselling.
- Men with complex general psychological problems.
- Men with complex psychosexual problems.
- Men and couples with relationship problems.
- Men or couples in whom there are complex ethical/legal issues.
- Men or couples who request such treatment as a preference.

How do you know whether the problem of ED is physical or psychological in origin?

Traditionally the following factors are considered to be important.

A physical cause is suggested if:

- The onset was gradual.
- Erectile failure is severe or complete.
- It is consistent and occurs regardless of the circumstances.
- There are no overt psychological factors.
- There is an identifiable physical cause.
A psychological cause is likely if:
- The onset was sudden without an obvious physical event.
- It varies according to the circumstances.
- There are overt psychological factors.
- There is no clear physical cause despite full assessment.

Can PDE5 inhibitors be taken by men on multiple antihypertensive drugs?

PDE5 inhibitors are not contraindicated in men taking antihypertensive drugs. Although there may be a slight reduction in blood pressure with PDE5 inhibitors, it is not clinically significant and there is not usually a synergistic effect. It is only nitrate drugs that may combine to produce a severe drop in blood pressure in some men, and this effect may only last for an hour or two.

Is treatment dangerous in the presence of heart disease?

No treatments are dangerous in the presence of heart disease provided the man is fit for sexual activity. Sexual activity is usually no more stressful physiologically than other normal everyday activities. It is important, however, to assess exercise tolerance in all men presenting with ED in order to assess the severity of any underlying vascular disease. Men with limited exercise tolerance should anyway be assessed by a cardiologist or other vascular specialist in order to optimize treatment of the underlying coronary or other artery disease. If fit for sexual activity, then men are safe to use any of the current treatments provided they are not taking nitrate drugs. If taking nitrates, then PDE5 inhibitors are contraindicated.

What about men on anticoagulant drugs such as warfarin?

There is no significant problem with oral treatments for ED. Intraurethral therapy may cause urethral bleeding and caution is required. Injection treatment may cause bruising but is safe to use provided care is taken and pressure applied to the injection site after injecting. Vacuum pumps are relatively contraindicated because of the risk of haematoma. If used very cautiously, however, they can be safe.

Is it worth changing men's antihypertensive drugs if ED is a problem?

This is a frequently asked question and many men will blame their antihypertensive drugs for their ED. ED is common anyway in hypertension whether treated or not. Increasingly, severe ED is associated with increasingly severe hypertension and the more severe the hypertension the more antihypertensive drugs are required. Naturally, there is therefore an association between ED and antihypertensive drugs regimes.

Experience suggests that there is little benefit to be had from altering antihypertensive drug regimes unless the man is certain there has been a direct temporal effect of a particular agent. Beta-blockers and diuretics are perhaps the worst culprits, and vasodilators and angiotensin-2 antagonists the least. This should be considered when starting antihypertensive drug regimes and men should be asked if they have any erection problems, and this should be monitored and explained if treatment changes are required for the hypertension.

What about peripheral vascular disease and ED?

This is an important association. Men with known peripheral vascular disease have a high prevalence of ED. Similarly, men with ED have a significant incidence of occult peripheral vascular disease and this may be severe. It is important to ask men about claudication and, if present, particularly proximally, they should be investigated with ultrasound. This is important not only to detect men with severe proximal major vessel disease, but also because occasionally correction of such vascular abnormalities can reverse the ED.

Misconceptions

- ED is a natural consequence of age and treatment is not warranted in the older man.

- ED is usually psychological in young men and they should be referred for counselling.
- Treatment is dangerous in the presence of heart disease.
- Sex is dangerous in the presence of heart disease.
- Treatment with multiple antihypertensive drugs is a contraindication to Viagra and other ED treatments.
- The NHS in the UK should not waste valuable resources on ED treatments.
- Men with ED should always be referred to a urologist for assessment.
- Men with ED should always be referred for psychosexual counselling.
- Penetrative sex is not always necessary for sexual satisfaction and men with ED should be advised to find alternatives.
- Men on anticoagulants should not use self-injection treatment for ED.
- Men with coronary artery disease, angina, myocardial infarct or coronary artery bypass surgery are not safe to use Viagra.

References

1. Craig A. *One in Ten*. London: Impotence Association, 1998.

2. Kinsey AC, Pomeroy WB, Martin CE. *Sexual Behaviour in the Human Male*. Philadelphia: WB Saunders, 1948.

3. Feldman HA, Goldstein I, Hatzichristou D *et al*. Impotence and its medical and psychological correlates: results of the Massachusetts Male Ageing Study: *J Urol* 1994; **151**: 54–61.

4. Masters WH, Johnson VE. *Human Sexual Inadequacy*. London: Churchill, 1970.

5. McCulloch DK, Campbell IW, Wu FC *et al*. The prevalence of diabetic impotence. *Diabetologia* 1980; **18**(4): 279–283.

6. Andersson KE, Wagener G. Physiology of penile erection. *Physiol Rev* 1995; **75**: 191–236.

7. Raijfer J, Aronson WJ, Bush PA *et al*. Nitric oxide as a mediator of the corpus cavernosum in response to non-cholinergic non-adrenergic neurotransmission. *New Engl J Med* 1992; **326**: 90–94.

8. Morales A, Heaton JPW, Carson CC. Andropause: misnomer for true clinical entity. *J Urol* 2000; **163**: 705-712.

9. Hohnquist F, Andersson KE, Fovaeus MN, Hedlmd H. Potassium channel openers for relaxation of isolated erectile tissue from rabbit. *J Urol* 1990; **144**: 146–151.

10. Kim YC, Kim JA, Hagan PO, Carson CC. Modulation of vasoactive intestinal polypeptide (VIP) mediated relaxation by nitric oxide and prostinoids in the rabbit corpus cavernosum. *J Urol* 1995; **153**: 807–810.

11. Iwanaga T, Hanyu S, Tainaki M. VIP and other bioactive substances involved in penile erection. *Biol Med Res* 1992; **2**: 71–73.

12. Kerfoot WW, Schwartz LB, Hagen PO, Carson CC. Characterization of contracting and relaxing agents in human and rabbit corpus cavernosum. *Surg Forum* 1991; **42**: 688–689.

13. Kim SC, Ooh MM. Norepinephrine involvement in response to intracorporeal injection of papaverine in psychogenic impotence. *J Urol* 1992; **147**: 1530–1532.

14. Brindley GS. Pilot experiments on the action of drugs injected into the human corpus cavernosum penis. *Br J Pharmacol* 1986; **87**: 405–500.

15. Rosen RC. Psychogenic erectile dysfunction: classification and management. *Urol Clin North Am* 2001; **28**: 269–278.

16. Shabsigh R, Klein LT, Seidman S *et al*. Increased incidence of depressive symptoms in men with erectile dysfunction. *Urology* 1998; **52**(5): 848–852.

17. Goldstein I. The mutually reinforcing triad of depressive symptoms, cardiovascular disease, and erectile dysfunction. *Am J Cardiol* 2000; **86**(2A): 41F–45F.

18. Tiefer L, Schuetz-Mueller D. Psychological issues in diagnosis and treatment of erectile disorders. *Urol Clin North Am* 1995; **22**(4): 767–773.

19. Chun J, Carson CC. Physician–patient dialog and clinical evaluation of erectile dysfunction. *Urol Clin North Am* 2001; **28**: 249–258.

20. McCulloch DK, Hosking DJ, Tobert A. A pragmatic approach to sexual dysfunction in diabetic men: psychosexual counseling. *Diabetic Med* 1986; **3**(5): 485–489.

21. O'Donoghue F. Psychological management of erectile dysfunction and related disorders. *Int J STD & AIDS* 1996; **7**(Suppl 3): 9–12.

22. Wylie KR. Male erectile disorder: characteristics and treatment choice of a longitudinal cohort study of men. *Int J Impotence Res* 1997; **9**(4): 217–224.

23. Araujo AB. Johannes CB. Feldman HA *et al*. Relation between psychosocial risk factors and incident erectile dysfunction: prospective results from the Massachusetts Male Aging Study. *Am J Epidemiol* 2000; **152**(6): 533–541.

24. Cavalini G. Minoxidil and capsacin: an association of transcutaneous active drugs for erection facilitation. *Int J Impotence Res* 1994; **6**: D71.

25. Heaton JPW, Morales A, Owen J *et al*. Topical glycerylternitate causes measurable penile arterial dilation in impotent men. *J Urol* 1990; **43**: 729–731.

26. Nunez BD, Andersson DC. Nitroglycerine ointment in the treatment of impotence. *J Urol* 1993; **150**: 1241–1243.

27. Cavalini G. Minoxidil versus nitroglycerin: prospective double-blind control trial in transcutaneous erection facilitation for organic impotence. *J Urol* 1991; **146**: 50–53.

28. Goldstein I, Payton TR, Schechter PJ. A double-blind, placebo-controlled, efficacy and safety study of topical gel formulation of 1% alprostadil (Topiglan) for the in-office treatment of erectile dysfunction. *Urology* 2001; **57**(2): 301–305.

29. McVary KT, Polepalle S, Riggi S. Topical prostaglandin E1 SEPA gel for the treatment of erectile dysfunction. *J Urol* 1999; **162**: 726–731.

30. Goldstein I, Lue TF, Padma-Nathan H *et al*. Oral sildenafil in the treatment of erectile dysfunction. Sildenafil Study Group. *New Engl J Med* 1998; **338**(20): 1397–1404.

31. Price DE. Sildenafil citrate (Viagra) efficacy in the treatment of erectile dysfunction in patients with common concomitant conditions. *Int J Clin Pract* 1999; **102**(Suppl): 21–23.

32. Kloner R, Brown M, et al. Effect of sildenafil in patients with erectile dysfunction taking antihypertensive therapy. Sildenafil Study Group. *Am J Hypertens* 2001; **14**:70–73

33.Brock GB *et al*. Efficacy and safety of tadalafil for the treatment of erectile dysfunction: results of integrated analyses. *J Urol* 2002; **168**(4 Pt 1):1332–1336.

34.Gbekor E et al. *EAU* 2002; **1** (suppl 1): 63.

35. Ballard SA, Gingell CJ *et al*. Effects of sildenafil on the relaxation of human corpus cavernosum tissue in vitro and on the activities of cyclic nucleotide phosphodiesterase isozymes. *J Urol* 1998; **159**(6):2164-2171.

36. Giuliano F, Allard J. Apomorphine SL (Uprima): preclinical and clinical experiences learned from the first central nervous system-acting ED drug. *Int J Impotence Res* 2002; **14**(Suppl 1): 553–556.

37. Padma-Nathan H, Hellstrom WJG, Kaiser FE *et al*. Treatment of men with erectile dysfunction with transurethral alprostadil. Medicated Urethral System for Erection (MUSE) Study Group. *New Engl J Med* 1997; **336**: 1–7.

38. Porst H. Transurethral alprostadil with MUSE versus intracavernous alprostadil: a comparative study in 103 patients with erectile dysfunction. *Int J Impotence Res* 1997; **9**: 187–192.

39. Fulgham PF *et al*. Disappointing initial results with transurethral alprostadil for erectile dysfunction in a urology practice setting. *J Urol* 1998; **160**: 2041–2046.

40. Shabsigh R, Padma-Nathan H, Gittleman M *et al*. Intracavernosal alprostadil alfadex is more efficacious, better tolerated and preferred over intraurethral alprostadil plus optional actis: a comparative, randomized, crossover, multicentre study. *Urology* 2000; **55**: 109–113.

41. Virag R. Intracavernosal injection of papaverine for erectile failure. *Lancet* 1982; **2**: 938.

42. Brindley GS. Cavernosal alpha blockade: a new treatment for investigating and treating erectile impotence. *Br J Psychol* 1983; **143**: 332–337.

43. Linet OI, Ogring FG. Efficacy in safety of intracavernosal alprostadil in men with erectile dysfunction. *New Engl J Med* 1996; **334**: 873–877.

44. Lee LM, Stevenson RW, Szasz G. Prostaglandin E-1 versus phentolamine–papaverine for the treatment of erectile impotence: a double-blind comparison. *J Urol* 1989; **141**: 549–550.

45. McMahon CG. A pilot study for the role of intracavernosal injection of vasoactive intestinal polypeptide (VIP) and phentolamine mesylate in the treatment of erectile dysfunction. *Int J Impotence Res* 1996; **8**: 233–236.

46. Kiely EA, Bloom SR, Williams G. Penile response to intracavernosal vasoactive intestinal polypeptide alone and in combination with other vasoactive agents. *Br J Urol* 1989; **64**: 191–194.

47. Gerstenberg TC, Metz T, Ottesen B, Fahrenkrug J. Intracavernous self-injection with vasoactive intestinal polypeptide and phentolamine in the management of erectile failure. *J Urol* 1992; **147**: 1277–1279.

48. Hermabessiere J, Costa CFP. Efficacy in safety assessment of intracavernous injection of moxisylyte in patients with erectile dysfunction: a double-blind placebo controlled study. *Int J Impotence Res* 1994; **6**: D147.

49. Buvat J, Costa P, Moralier D *et al*. Double-blind multicenter study comparing alprostadil alpha cyclodextrin with moxisylyte chlorohydrate in patients with chronic erectile dysfunction. *J Urol* 1998; **159**: 116–119.

50. Vick RN, Benevides M, Patel M *et al.* The efficacy, safety and tolerability of intracavernous PNU-83757 for the treatment of erectile dysfunction. *J Urol* 2002; **167**(6): 2618–2623.

51. Shabsigh R, Padma-Nathan H, Gittleman M *et al.* Intracavernous alprostadil alfadex (EDEX/VIRIDAL) is effective and safe in patients with erectile dysfunction after failing sildenafil (Viagra). *Urology* 2000; **55**(4): 477–480.

52. Mydlo JH, Volpe MA, MacChia RJ. Results from different patient populations using combined therapy with alprostadil and sildenafil: predictors of satisfaction. *BJU Int* 2000; **86**(4): 469–473.

53. Cookson MS, Nadig PW. Long-term results with vacuum constriction devices. *J Urol* 1993; **149**(2): 290–294.

54. Turner LA, Althof SE, Levine SB *et al.* External vacuum devices in the treatment of erectile dysfunction: a one year study of sexual and psychosocial impact. *J Sex Marital Ther* 1991; **17**(2): 81–93.

55. Carson CC. Penile prostheses. In: Kirby RS, Carson CC, Webster GD, editors. *Impotence: Diagnosis and Management of Male Erectile Dysfunction.* Oxford: Butterworth-Heinemann, 1991; pp. 167–176.

56. Small MP, Carrion HM, Gordon JA. Small carrion penile prosthesis: a new implant for the management of impotence. *Urology* 1975; **5**: 479–486.

57. Scott FB, Bradley WE, Timm DW. Management of erectile impotence: use of implantable inflatable prosthesis. *Urology* 1973; **2**: 80–83.

58. Carson CC, Mulcahy JJ, Govier FE. Efficacy, safety, and patient satisfaction outcomes of the AMS 700CX inflatable penile prosthesis: results of a long term multicenter study. *J Urol* 2000; **164**: 376–380.

59. Carson CC. Reconstructive surgery using urological prostheses. *Curr Opin Urol* 1999; **9**: 233–239.

60. Mulcahy JJ. Long term experience with salvage of infected penile implants. *J Urol* 2000; **163**: 481–482.

61. Wilson SK, Cleves MA, Delk JR. Comparison of mechanical reliability of original and enhanced mentor alpha-1 penile prosthesis. *J Urol* 1999; **162**: 715–718.

62. Goldstein I, Newman L, Baum N *et al*. Safety and efficacy outcome of mentor alpha-1 inflatable penile prosthesis implantation for impotence treatment. *J Urol* 1997; **157**: 833–839.

63. Kerfoot WW, Carson CC, Donaldson JT, Kliewer MA. Investigation of vascular changes following penile vein ligation. *J Urol* 1994; **153**: 884–887.

64. Goldwasser B, Carson CC, Braun SD, McCann RL. Impotence due to the pelvic steal syndrome: treatment by iliac transluminal angioplasty. *J Urol* 1985; **133**: 860–861.

65. Goldstein I. Arterial revascularization procedures. *Semin Urol* 1986; **4**: 252–258.

66. Berger R, Billups K, Brock G *et al*. Report of the American Foundation for Urologic Disease (AFUD) Thought Leader Panel for evaluation and treatment of priapism. *Int J Impotence Res* 2001; **13**(Suppl 5): S39–S43.

67. Chan PT, Begin LR, Arnold D *et al*. Priapism secondary to penile metastasis: a report of two cases and a review of the literature. *J Surg Oncol* 1998; **68**: 51–59.

68. Eland IA, van der Lei J, Stricker BH, Sturkenboom MJ. Incidence of priapism in the general population. *Urology* 2001; **57**: 970–972.

69. Fowler JE Jr, Koshy M, Strub M, Chinn SK. Priapism associated with the sickle cell hemoglobinopathies: prevalence, natural history and sequelae. *J Urol* 1991; **145**: 65–68.

70. Mantadakis E, Cavender JD, Rogers ZR *et al*. Prevalence of priapism in children and adolescents with sickle cell anemia. *J Pediatr Hematol Oncol* 1999; **21**: 518–522.

71. Compton MT, Miller AH. Priapism associated with conventional and atypical antipsychotic medications: a review. *J Clin Psychiat* 2001; **62**: 362–366.

72. Altman AL, Seftel AD, Brown SL, Hampel N. Cocaine associated priapism. *J Urol* 1999; **161**: 1817–1818.

73. Bschleipfer TH, Hauck EW, Diemer TH *et al*. Heparin-induced priapism. *Int J Impotence Res* 2001; **13**: 357–359.

74. Hebuterne X, Frere AM, Bayle J, Rampal P. Priapism in a patient treated with total parenteral nutrition. *J Parenter Enteral Nutr* 1992; **16**: 171–174.

75. Kachhi PN, Henderson SO. Priapism after androstenedione intake for athletic performance enhancement. *Ann Emerg Med* 2000; **35**: 391–393.

76. Whalen RK, Whitcomb RW, Crowley WF Jr, McGovern FJ. Priapism in hypogonadal men receiving gonadotropin releasing hormone. *J Urol* 1991; **145**: 1051–1052.

77. Zargooshi J. Priapism as a complication of high dose testosterone therapy in a man with hypogonadism. *J Urol* 2000; **163**: 907.

78. Keoghane SR, Sullivan ME, Miller MA. The aetiology, pathogenesis and management of priapism. *BJU Int* 2002; **90**(2): 149–154.

79. Broderick GA, Gordon D, Hypolite J, Levin RM. Anoxia and corporal smooth muscle dysfunction: a model for ischemic priapism. *J Urol* 1994; **151**: 259–262.

80. Bastuba MD, Saenz de Tejada I, Dinlenc CZ *et al*. Arterial priapism: diagnosis, treatment and long-term follow-up. *J Urol* 1994; **151**: 1231–1237.

81. Pautler SE, Brock GB. Priapism. From Priapus to the present time. *Urol Clin North Am* 2001; **28**: 391–403. A very thorough review of all subtypes of priapism.

82. Lee M, Cannon B, Sharifi R. Chart for preparation of dilutions of alpha-adrenergic agonists for intracavernous use in treatment of priapism. *J Urol* 1995; **153**: 1182–1183.

83. Futral AA, Witt MA. A closed system for corporeal irrigation in the treatment of refractory priapism. *Urology* 1995; **46**: 403–404.

84. Levine LA, Guss SP. Gonadotropin-releasing hormone analogues in the treatment of sickle cell anemia-associated priapism. *J Urol* 1993; **150**: 475–477.

85. Steinberg J, Eyre RC. Management of recurrent priapism with epinephrine self-injection and gonadotropin-releasing hormone analogue. *J Urol* 1995; **153**: 152–153.

86. Hakim LS, Kulaksizoglu H, Mulligan R *et al*. Evolving concepts in the diagnosis and treatment of arterial high flow priapism. *J Urol* 1996; **155**: 541–548.

87. Ciampalini S, Savoca G, Buttazzi L *et al*. High-flow priapism: treatment and long-term follow-up. *Urology* 2002; **59**: 110–113.

88. Lischer GH, Nehra A. New advances in Peyronie's disease. *Curr Opin Urol* 2001; **11**(6): 631–636.

89. Noss MB, Day NS, Christ GJ, Melman A. The genetics and immunology of Peyronie's disease. *Int J Impotence Res* 2000; **12**(Suppl 4): S127–S132.

90. Carson CC, Lue T, Levine L *et al*. Symposium on Peyronie's disease, 12 April 1997. *Int J Impotence Res* 1998; **10**(2): 121–122.

91. Carrieri MP, Serraino D, Palmiotto F *et al*. A case-control study on risk factors for Peyronie's disease. *J Clin Epidemiol* 1998; **51**(6): 511–515.

92. Carson CC. Potassium para-aminobenzoate for the treatment of Peyronie's disease: is it effective? *Techniques Urol* 1997; **3**(3): 135–139.

93. Hellstrom WJ, Bivalacqua TJ. Peyronie's disease: etiology, medical, and surgical therapy. *J Androl* 2000; **21**(3): 347–354.

94. Levine LA. Advances in the medical therapy of Peyronie's disease: a brief review. *Int J Impotence Res* 1998; **10**(2): 123–124.

95. Chun JL, McGregor A, Krishnan R, Carson CC. A comparison of dermal and cadaveric pericardial grafts in the modified Horton–Devine procedure for Peyronie's disease. *J Urol* 2001; **166**(1): 185–188.

96. Carson CC. Penile prosthesis implantation in the treatment of Peyronie's disease and erectile dysfunction. *Int J Impotence Res* 2000; **12**(Suppl 4): S122–S126.

97. Carson CC, Mulcahy JJ, Govier FE. Efficacy, safety and patient satisfaction outcomes of the AMS 700CX inflatable penile prosthesis: results of a long-term multicenter study. AMS 700CX Study Group.

98. Price D, O'Malley BP, James MA *et al*. Why are impotent diabetic men not being treated? *Pract Diabet* 1991; **8**: 10–11.

99. Stief CG. Is there a common pathophysiology of erectile dysfunction and how does this relate to new pharmacotherapies? *Int J Impotence Res* 2002; **14**(Suppl 1): S11–S16.

100. Wespes E. Smooth muscle pathology and erectile dysfunction. *Int J Impotence Res* 2002; **14**(Suppl 1): S17–S21.

101. Burchardt M, Burchardt T, Baer L *et al.* Hypertension is associated with severe erectile dysfunction. *J Urol* 2000; **164**: 1188–1191.

102. Greenstein A, Chen J, Miller H *et al.* Does severity of ischemic coronary disease correlate with erectile function? *Int J Impotence Res* 1997; **9**: 123–126.

103. Hellerstein HK. *Arch Int med* 1970, **125**: 987–999

104. Muller JE, Mittleman A, Maclure M *et al.* Triggering myocardial infarction by sexual activity. Low absolute risk and prevention by regular physical exertion. Determinants of Myocardial Infarction Onset Study investigators. *J Am Med Assoc* 1996; **275**: 1405–1409.

105. Wilson PK, Farday PS, Froelicher V, Editors. *Cardiac Rehabilitation: Adult Fitness and Exercise Testing.* Philadelphia: Lea & Fabiger, 1981.

106. Jackson G, Betteridge J, Dean J *et al.* A systematic approach to erectile dysfunction in the cardiovascular patient: a consensus statement. *Int J Clin Pract* 1999; **53**: 445–451.

107. Master VA, Turek PJ. Ejaculatory physiology and dysfunction. *Urol Clin North Am* 2001; **28**(2): 363–375.

108. Waldinger MD, Zwinderman AH, Olivier B. SSRIs and ejaculation: a double-blind, randomized, fixed-dose study with paroxetine and citalopram. *J Clin Psychopharmacol* 2001; **21**(6): 556–560.

109. Blanker MH, Bosch JL, Groeneveld FP *et al.* Erectile and ejaculatory dysfunction in a community-based sample of men 50 to 78 years old: prevalence, concern, and relation to sexual activity. *Urology* 2001; **57**(4): 763–768.

110. Laumann EO, Paik A, Rosen RC. The epidemiology of erectile dysfunction: results from the National Health and Social Life Survey. *Int J Impotence Res* 1999; **11**(Suppl 1): S60–S64.

111. Rowland DL, Strassberg DS, de Gouveia Brazao CA, Slob AK. Ejaculatory latency and control in men with premature ejaculation: an analysis across sexual activities using multiple sources of information. *J Psychosom Res* 2000; **48**(1): 69–77.

112. Waldinger MD, Zwinderman AH, Olivier B. Antidepressants and ejaculation: a double-blind, randomized, placebo-controlled, fixed-dose study with paroxetine, sertraline, and nefazodone. *J Clin Psychopharmacol* 2001; **21**(3): 293–297.

113. McMahon CG, Touma K. Treatment of premature ejaculation with paroxetine hydrochloride as needed: 2 single-blind placebo controlled crossover studies. *J Urol* 1999; **161**(6): 1826–1830.

114. Goldmeier D, Lamba H. Assessment of as needed use of pharmacotherapy and the pause-squeeze technique in premature ejaculation by Abdel-Hamid *et al*. *Int J Impotence Res* 2001; **13**(4): 252.

115. Morales A. Developmental status of topical therapies for erectile and ejaculatory dysfunction. *Int J Impotence Res* 2000; **12**(Suppl 4): S80–S85.

116. Motofei IG. Re: Treatment of premature ejaculation with paroxetine hydrochloride as needed: 2 single-blind placebo controlled crossover studies. *J Urol* 2002; **168**(4, Pt 1): 1508–1509.

117. Ohl DA, Wolf LJ, Menge AC *et al*. Electroejaculation and assisted reproductive technologies in the treatment of anejaculatory infertility. *Fertil Steril* 2001; **76**(6): 1249–1255.

118. Biering-Sorensen F, Sonksen J. Sexual function in spinal cord lesioned men. *Spinal Cord* 2001; **39**(9): 455–470.

119. Rosen RC, Lane RM, Menza M. Effects of SSRIs on sexual function: a critical review. *J Clin Psychopharmacol* 1999; **19**(1): 67–85.

120. Furuya S, Ogura H, Saitoh N *et al*. Hematospermia: an investigation of the bleeding site and underlying lesions. *Int J Urol* 1999; **6**(11): 539–547.

121. Munkelwitz R, Krasnokutsky S, Lie J *et al*. Current perspectives on hematospermia: a review. *J Androl* 1997; **18**(1): 6–14.

122. Wagner G, Lacy S, Lewis R. Buccal phentolamine: a pilot trial for male erectile dysfunction at three separate clinics. *Int J Impotence Res* 1994; **6**: D78.

123. Schenk G, Melman A, Christ G. Gene therapy: future therapy for erectile dysfunction. *Curr Urol Rep* 2001; **2**(6): 480–487.

124. Heaton JPW, Adams MA, Morales A. Therapeutic taxonomy of treatments for erectile dysfunction: an evolutionary imperative. *Int J Impotence Res* 1997; **9**: 115–121.

125. O'Leary MP, Fowler FJ, Lenderking WR *et al*. A brief male sexual function inventory for urology. *Urology* 1993; **56**: 697–706.

126. MacDonagh R, Ewings M, Porter T. The effect of erectile dysfunction on quality of life: psychometric testing of a new quality of life measure for patients with erectile dysfunction. *J Urol* 2002; **167**(1): 212–217.

127. Zigmund AS, Snaith RP. The Hospital Anxiety and Depression Scale. *Acta Psychiat Scand* 1983; **67**: 361–370.

128. Beck AT, Rush AJ, Shaw BF. *Cognitive Therapy of Depression*. New York: Guilford Press, 1979.

129. Goldberg D. *Manual of the General Health Questionnaire*. Windsor: NFER, 1978.

Appendix 1 – Drugs

Drug	Trade name	Preparation	Strength
Alprostadil	Caverject Injection	Intercavernosal injection	5, 10, 20, 40 mcg
	Caverject Dual Chamber Injection	Intercavernosal injection	10, 20 mcg
	Viridal Duo	Intercavernosal injection	10, 20, 40 mcg
	MUSE Urethral Application	Urethral application	125, 250, 500 mcg, 1 mg
Apomorphine	Uprima	Sublingual tablet	2, 3 mg

Doses used in ED	Comments	Side-effects
2.5 mcg first dose, 5–7.5 mcg second dose depending on response then increasing by 5–10 mcg steps to obtain dose suitable for producing erection lasting <1 hour; usual range 5–20 mcg (max. 60 mcg; max. frequency once daily and 3 doses/week)	Contraindicated in predisposition to prolonged erection (e.g. sickle cell anaemia, multiple myeloma, leukaemia), patients with penile implants, conditions where sexual activity is medically inadvisable	Penile pain, priapism, injection site reactions haematoma, haemosiderin deposits, penile rash, penile oedema, penile fibrosis, haemorrhage, inflammation, other local reactions (urethral burning or bleeding, penile warmth or numbness, penile or urinary tract infection, irritation, sensitivity, phimosis, pruritus, erythema, venous leak, abnormal ejaculation), systemic effects (testicular pain and swelling, changes in micturition, dry mouth, hypotension or hypertension, fainting, rapid pulse, vasodilatation, chest pain, supraventricular extrasystole, peripheral vascular disorder, dizziness, weakness, localized pain, headache, influenza-like syndrome
2.5 mcg first dose then increasing by 2.5–5 mcg steps to obtain dose suitable for producing erection lasting <1 hour; usual range 10–20 mcg (max. 40 mcg; max. frequency once daily and 2–3 doses/week)		
250 mcg first dose then adjust according to response; usual range 0.125–1 mg (max. frequency 2 times/day and 7 doses/week)	Urethral application contraindicated in urethral stricture, severe hypospadia, severe curvature, balanitis, urethritis; caution in anatomical deformations of the penis	
Sexual activity (max. 2 mg 20 minute before 3 mg; min. of 8 hours between doses)	Recent myocardial infarction, severe unstable angina, severe heart failure or hypotension, conditions where sexual activity is medically inadvisable; caution in hepatic and renal impairment (reduce dose), uncontrolled hypertension, hypotension, elderly, anatomical deformation of the penis (e.g. angulation, cavernosal fibrosis, Peyronie's disease)	Nausea, headache, dizziness, yawning, drowsiness, rhinitis, pharyngitis, cough, flushing, taste disturbance, sweating

Drug	Trade name	Preparation	Strength
Sildenafil	Viagra	Tablet	25, 50, 100 mg
Tadalafil	Cialis	Tablet	10, 20 mg
Vardenalfil	Levitra	Tablet	5, 10, 20 mg

Doses used in ED	Comments	Side-effects
50 mg (elderly 25 mg) 1 hour before sexual activity; range 25–100 mg (max. 100 mg; max. frequency once daily)	Contraindicated in patients taking nitrates, conditions in which vasodilatation or sexual activity is inadvisable, recent stroke or myocardial infarction, hypotension, hereditary retinal disorders; caution in cardiovascular disease, anatomical deformation of the penis (e.g. angulation, cavernosal fibrosis, Peyronie's disease), predisposition to prolonged erection (e.g. sickle cell anaemia, multiple myeloma, leukaemia), reduce dose in hepatic and renal impairment	Dyspepsia, vomiting, headache, flushing, dizziness, visual disturbances and increased intraocular pressure, nasal congestion, hypersensitivity reactions, priapism
10 mg 30 minutes–12 hours before sexual activity (range 10–20 mg, max frequency once daily)	Contraindicated in patients taking nitrates, conditions in which sexual activity is inadvisable (cardiac disease), men under 18 years, women; caution in patients taking ketoconazole, itraconazole, erythromycin, clarithromycin or protease inhibitors	Headache, dyspepsia, dizziness, flushing, nasal congestion, back pain, myalgia
10 mg (elderly, mild or moderate hepatic impairment, severe renal impairment 5 mg) 25minutes–1 hour before sexual activity (range 5–20 mg, max frequency once daily)	Contraindicated in patients taking nitrates, conditions in which vasodilatation or sexual activity is inadvisable (e.g. severe cardiac disease), severe hepatic impairment, end stage renal disease requiring dialysis, hypotension, recent stroke or myocardial infarction, hypotension, unstable angina, hereditary retinal degenerative disorders, concurrent use of ritonavir, indinavir, ketoconazole, itraconazole, women; caution in cardiovascular disease , anatomical deformation of the penis, predisposition to priapism (e.g. sickle cell anaemia, multiple myeloma, leukaemia), bleeding disorders, active peptic ulceration	Flushing, headache, dyspepsia, nausea, dizziness, rhinitis, hypertension, photosensitivity reactions, abnormal vision, hypertonia, hypotension, syncope, erectile disturbance, priapism (at doses higher than max recommended)

Appendix 2 – Useful Addresses and Websites

The Impotence Association (UK) (www.impotence.org.uk)
PO Box 10296,
London SW17 9WH, UK
Tel.: +44 (0)20 8767 7791

The Impotence Association is a charitable organization which was set up to help sufferers of impotence (erectile dysfunction) and their partners, and to raise awareness of the condition amongst both the public and the medical profession.

Impotence Institute of America (IIA)
8201 Corporate Drive, Suite 320
Landover, MD 20785, USA
Tel.: +1 800 669 1603

The Impotence Institute of America (IIA), a division of the Impotence World Association, is a non-profit organization dedicated to education about impotence. The IIA provides information on the causes, impact and treatments on this topic. It also publishes a quarterly newsletter on impotence topics and helps sponsor support groups for men with ED and their partners.

American Urological Association (AUA) (www.auanet.org)
1120 North Charles Street
Baltimore, MD 21201-5559, USA
Tel.: +1 410 727 1100

The AUA is a non-profit professional organization that represents urologists and scientists in the field of urology. The AUA strives to promote the highest standards of urological care through education, research and formulation of healthcare policy.

British Association of Urological Surgeons
(www.baus.org.uk)
The Royal College of Surgeons of England
35/43 Lincoln's Inn Fields
London WC2A 3PE
Tel.: +44 (0)20 7869 6950

International Society for Sexual and Impotence Research
(ISSIR) (www.urolog.nl/artsen/isir)
ISSIR Secretariet
Status Plus
PO Box 97
3950 AB Maarn
The Netherland
Tel.: +31 343 443 888

The ISSIR was founded in 1982 for the purpose of promoting research and exchange of knowledge for the clinical entity, impotence, throughout the international scientific community. The principal orientation of the ISSIR is toward the basic science of erection, defects in the erectile mechanism, and the clinical aspects of diagnosis and treatment of erectile dysfunction.

British Society for Sexual Medicine (BSSM)
(www.bssm.org.uk)

The British Society for Sexual Medicine (BSSM) was founded in 1997. The principal orientation of the BSSM is toward the basic science of sexual function and dysfunction, and the clinical aspects of diagnosis and treatment of sexual problems in both men and women.

European Society for Sexual and Impotence Research
(ESSIR) (www.essir.com)
Reichskanzler Str. 8
22609 Hamburg
Germany
Tel.: +49 40 350 159 16

American Association of Sex Educators, Counselors and Therapists (AASECT) (www.aasect.org)
P.O. Box 5488
Richmond, VA 23220-0488, USA

The AASECT represents a wide range of health professionals who are interested in promoting understanding of human sexuality and sexual behaviour.

British Association for Sexual and Relationship Therapy (BASRT) (www.basrt.org.uk)
PO Box 13686
London SW20 9ZH, UK
Tel.: +44 (0)20 8543 2707

Lists of and information about therapists in the UK.

Prostate Health (www.prostatehealth.com)

This site offers advice from urologists and primary care practitioners about conditions affecting prostate health.

American Diabetes Association (ADA) (www.diabetes.org)
National Call Centre
1701 North Beauregard Street
Alexandria, VA 22311, USA
Tel.: +1-800 342 2383

The ADA is the USA's leading non-profit health organization providing diabetes research, information and advocacy. It offers many free publications for people with diabetes, including several brochures and articles on men's sexual health.

Diabetes UK (www.diabetes.org.uk)
10 Parkway
London NW1 7AA, UK
Tel.: +44 (0)20 7424 1000

Diabetes UK is the largest organisation in the UK working for people with diabetes, funding research, campaigning and helping people live with the condition and its complications.

Appendix 3 – Medical Suppliers and Manufacturers of Vacuum Devices for Erectile Dysfunction

Osbon Medical
91 Weston Park
London N9 9PR, UK
Tel.: +44 (0)20 8340 7311

Farnhurst Medical
Unit 11, Alford Craft and Business Centre
Loxwood, Alford
Surrey GU6 8HP, UK
Tel.: +44 (0)1403 753 838

Eurosurgical Ltd
Merrow Business Centre
Guilford
Surrey GU4 7WA, UK
Tel.: +44 (0)1483 456 007

Vetco UK
PO Box 87
Bexhill-on-sea
East Sussex TN39 4ZE, UK
Tel.: +44 (0)1424 848 111

Genesis Medical
Linton House
39–51 Highgate Road
London NW5 1RT, UK
Tel.: +44 (0)20 7284 2824

Mediwatch
Swift House
Cosford lane
Swift Valley Industrial Estate
Rugby
Warwickshire CV21 1QN, UK
Tel.: +44 (0)1788 547 888

Healthcare 2000
Duncan House
Duncan Street
Leeds LS1 6DL, UK
Tel.: +44 (0)1904 607 477

Owen Mumford
Brook Hill
Woodstock
Oxford OX20 1TU, UK
Tel.: +44 (0)1993 812 433

Appendix 4 – Questionnaires for Use in Assessment of Sexual Dysfunction

IIEF: International Index of Erectile Function (Erectile Domain)

[Print out questionnaire]

SHIM: Sexual Health Inventory for Men

[Print out questionnaire]

Other available questionnaires:

Male Sexual Function Questionnaire[125]

ED-EqoL Quality of Life Questionnaire[126] The effect of erectile dysfunction on quality of life: psychometric testing of a new quality of life measure for patients with erectile dysfunction.

HADS: Hospital Anxiety and Depression Scale[127]

BDI: Beck's Depression Inventory[128]

GHQ: General Health Questionnaire[129]

INDEX

Please note that as the subject of this book is erectile dysfunction, entries under this term have been kept to a minimum, readers are advised to seek more specific entries. This index is presented in letter-by-letter order, whereby spaces and hyphens in main entries are excluded from the alphabetization process. Page numbers followed by the letters 'f' and 't' refer to figures and tables respectively.